# NEUROLOGICAL EMERGENCIES IN MEDICAL PRACTICE: A Handbook for the Non-specialist

The purpose of this book is to provide a concise, symptom-oriented text on the diagnosis and management of neurological emergencies for the front-line medical practitioner. This might be a family doctor or a hospital doctor working in an accident and emergency department, or whoever first treats the patient. Written by neurologists and neurosurgeons from Britain and the USA who have daily first-hand experience of the subjects they discuss, the aim of the book is to be essentially practical and it should be of immediate value to a wide range of clinicians.

Edited by David Bowsher, Reader in the Department of Neurological Science at the University of Liverpool.

# Neurological Emergencies in Medical Practice:

A Handbook for the Non-specialist

Edited by
DAVID BOWSHER

CROOM HELM
London & Sydney

© 1988 David Bowsher
Croom Helm Ltd, Provident House,
Burrell Row, Beckenham, Kent BR3 1AT
Croom Helm Australia, 44–50 Waterloo Road,
North Ryde, 2113, New South Wales

British Library Cataloguing in Publication Data

Neurological emergencies in medical practice:
    a handbook for the non-specialist
    1. Nervous system — Diseases
    I. Bowsher, David
    ISBN 0-7099-5013-6


Distributed exclusively in the USA by Sheridan House Inc.,
145 Palisade Street, Dobbs Ferry NY 10522

Filmset by Mayhew Typesetting, Bristol, England
Printed and bound in Great Britain by
Biddles Ltd, Guildford and King's Lynn

# Contents

# Preface

Neurology has a reputation for being 'difficult' among the majority of doctors who do not practise it in one of its medical or surgical forms. Whether this is because the time devoted to it in the medical curriculum is inadequate, or because (God forbid!) its practitioners behave like High Priests exercising a mystery beyond the ken of lesser mortals must be left to others to decide. Naturally, the editor and authors of this book incline to the former explanation

In addition to a perhaps inadequate early training, neurological/neurosurgical cases are relatively rare among the mass of pathology encountered by the average community or hospital doctor in his or her daily experience. For example, many general practitioners recount that they have *never* seen a case of 'thalamic syndrome'; yet this author currently has over 40 attending his clinic — which probably means that it is commoner than motor neurone disease (amyotrophic lateral sclerosis).

This small book, which will hopefully fit into the glovebox of a car if not into the pocket, has been conceived in order to demystify and explain those many and various neurological emergencies across which any doctor may come any day. What we have set out to do is, first, to describe how to recognise/diagnose the various conditions, and secondly how to deal with them.

So this is essentially a practical manual. If you think any part of it could be improved, please write and tell us how!

**David Bowsher**
Department of Neurological Sciences
University of Liverpool

# Contributors

Michael S. Aldrich, M.D., Assistant Professor of Neurology, University of Michigan Medical Center, Ann Arbor, Michigan

Thomas K. Aldrich, M.D., Assistant Professor, Division of Pulmonary Medicine, Department of Internal Medicine, Montefiore Medical Center, New York

Peter G. Blain, B.Med.Sci., M.R.C.P., C.Biol., M.I.Biol., Professor of Occupational Health and Hygiene, University of Newcastle upon Tyne

Lance Blumhardt, B.Sci., M.D., F.R.A.C.P., Senior Lecturer in Neurology, Department of Neurological Sciences, University of Liverpool, and Honorary Consultant Neurologist, Mersey Regional Health Authority, Walton Hospital, Liverpool

David Bowsher, M.A., M.D., Ph.D., M.R.C.P.Ed., M.R.C.Path., Reader (Clinical) in Neurological Sciences, University of Liverpool

Gordon F.G. Findlay, B.Sc., M.B., Ch.B., F.R.C.S., Consultant Neurosurgeon and Clinical Lecturer, University of Liverpool

Daniel F. Hanley, M.D., Director of Neurosciences Intensive Care Unit, The Johns Hopkins Hospital, Baltimore, Maryland

Simon P. Harding, M.B., Ch.B., F.R.C.S., Lecturer in Ophthalmology, University of Liverpool, and Honorary Senior Registrar, St Paul's Eye Hospital, Liverpool

Russell J.M. Lane, B.Sc., M.D., M.R.C.P., Senior Registrar in Neurology, Charing Cross Hospital, London

A. David Mendelow, M.B., B.Ch., Ph.D., F.R.C.S.Ed., F.R.C.S.Ed. (Surgical Neurology), Reader in Neurosurgery, University of Newcastle upon Tyne, and Honorary Consultant, Newcastle General Hospital

Bruce Moffatt, M.D., Departments of Neurosurgery, Neurology, and Anesthesia Critial Care Medicine, The Johns Hopkins Hospital, Baltimore, Maryland

John R. Patten, B.Sc., M.B., F.R.C.P., Consultant Neurologist, Royal Surrey Hospital, Guildford, Surrey

Peter A.G. Sandercock, B.A., D.M., M.R.C.P., Lecturer in Neurology, University of Liverpool

John B. Selhorst, M.D., Professor and Chairman, Department of Neurology, St. Louis University School of Medicine, St. Louis, Missouri

# 1

# How to Recognise and Examine a Neurological Emergency

John B. Selhorst

## INTRODUCTION

The relevance of a careful neurological assessment is evident in population-based statistics. The prevalence rate for diseases affecting the nervous system in the United States is 9.5%, and new cases are encountered at an annual incidence of 2.5% (Kurtzke, 1984). More importantly, nearly 2% of these cases are acutely disabling and potentially very serious illnesses. Thus, the general practitioner should regularly expect to be confronted with acute neurological disorders.

Not infrequently the non-neurologist's recollections of neuroanatomical pathways and eponymic clinical signs are vague. A reliable and orderly clinical method to classify a neurological illness and begin its management is needed. To tackle an evolving neurological emergency, the time-tested methodology to divide and conquer is employed and accomplished in the following steps. First, the presence of a neurological disorder is acknowledged. Secondly, the process is assigned to either the central or peripheral nervous system or both and localised within the anatomical subdivisions of these systems. Thirdly, the pathology is characterised by the temporal evolution, type and distribution of symptoms and signs. Fourthly, the site and character of the disturbance are confirmed by the neurological examination and appropriately selected diagnostic studies. Finally, the accuracy of this estimation is verified by the response to treatment and course of the illness. The following commentary details how these specific steps are achieved, and an outline of the orderly process is illustrated in the accompanying figure (Figure 1.1).

1

**Figure 1.1:** Schematic history and physical for neurologic emergency

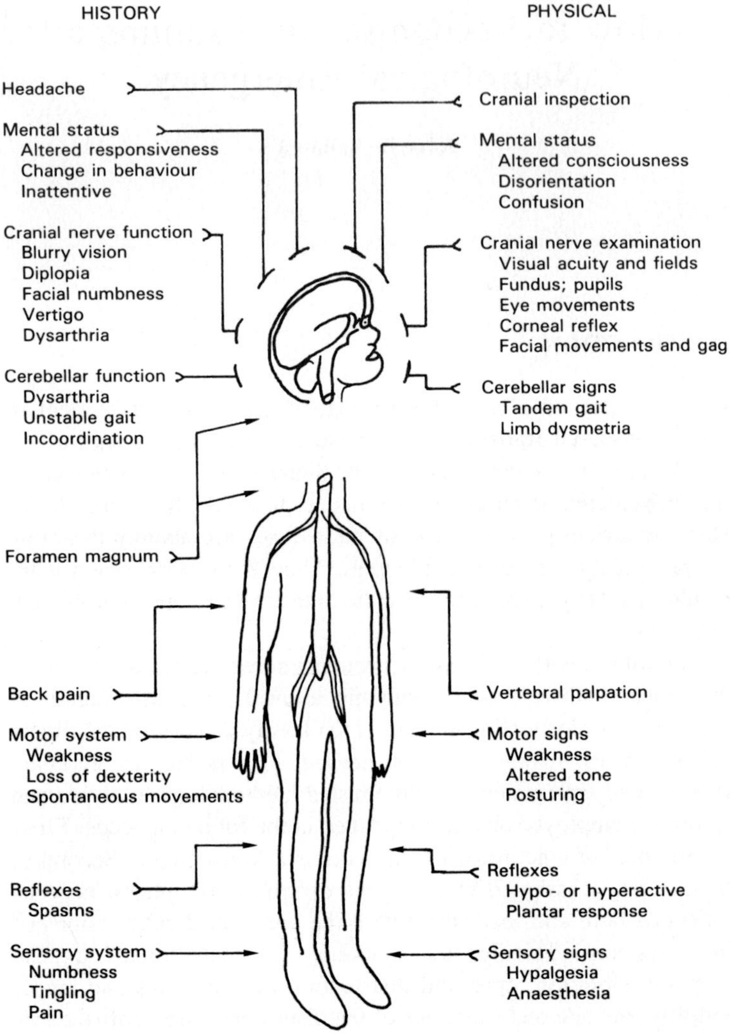

HISTORY                                    PHYSICAL

Headache                                   Cranial inspection

Mental status                              Mental status
  Altered responsiveness                     Altered consciousness
  Change in behaviour                        Disorientation
  Inattentive                                Confusion

Cranial nerve function                     Cranial nerve examination
  Blurry vision                              Visual acuity and fields
  Diplopia                                   Fundus; pupils
  Facial numbness                            Eye movements
  Vertigo                                    Corneal reflex
  Dysarthria                                 Facial movements and gag

Cerebellar function                        Cerebellar signs
  Dysarthria                                 Tandem gait
  Unstable gait                              Limb dysmetria
  Incoordination

Foramen magnum

Back pain                                  Vertebral palpation

Motor system                               Motor signs
  Weakness                                   Weakness
  Loss of dexterity                          Altered tone
  Spontaneous movements                      Posturing

Reflexes                                   Reflexes
  Spasms                                     Hypo- or hyperactive
                                             Plantar response

Sensory system                             Sensory signs
  Numbness                                   Hypalgesia
  Tingling                                   Anaesthesia
  Pain

2

## THE HISTORY

The clinician's recognition of a neurological disorder begins with the personal introduction. No single moment yields more useful information to the neurological assessment. The chief functions of the nervous system — cognition, locomotion and sensory detection — are immediately evident for inspection. For example, the patient with acute pain or crippled movements is readily apparent. Because the nervous system is the control centre for many complex and highly developed functions, close inspection commonly discloses an abnormality. The mental status examination commences as the physician introduces him- or herself and verifies the identity of the patient. To relax patients and better understand the personal significance of their complaints, it is useful to inquire about their occupation, e.g. roofer, salesman, housewife, secretary. The level of attention, conveyance of affect, choice of language and lucidity of verbal expression are noted and should be directly and further pursued if other than normal. A mental pause to assess the appropriateness of the patient's appearance, behaviour and comfort is rewarding in providing clues to a cerebral malfunction.

After the introduction, the primary complaint is sought. The earnest clinician listens critically to the patient's concerns and choice of words. Further questioning as to just how the symptom complex affects the patient's customary lifestyle and habits often assists in clarifying the presence and magnitude of sensory disturbances, motor deficits or intellectual impairment. Thus, an acute illness striking the nervous system is readily identified.

Next, by employing a series of skilful questions, the clinician establishes which part of the nervous system is disturbed. Attention is especially given to the principal location and distribution of pain as well as the functional complaints. A useful anatomical landmark for the assignment of symptoms is the foramen magnum. This is because the nature of the diseases affecting the nervous system above and below this opening in the skull and the subsequent choice of diagnostic tests to confirm the neurological disorder are so different. The following exposition pertains to symptoms of disorders above the foramen magnum.

Headache results from the stimulation of pain fibres found either in the scalp or contained in the meninges and its blood vessels. Most headaches involving the scalp are due to muscle contraction or migraine-associated changes in the blood vessels. These conditions are emergent in so far as they demand relief. Exceptions among extracranial headaches are those conditions associated with inflammation or arteritis. Intracranial processes causing acute headache are meningeal infections or disorders resulting in sudden stretching or compression of the meninges such as haemorrhage or hydrocephalus. The headache is commonly aching in quality and either focal or generalised. Pain in the posterior neck is an additional complaint of patients with cerebellar or lower brainstem disease. Intracranial headaches are ordinarily constant or progressive over time, which distinguishes them from the pain-free, episodic intervals that are common with migraine and tension headaches. Vomiting is a less specific sign of intracranial disease but occurs in patients with acute processes involving an increase in pressure or inflammation extending into the ventricular cavity. Presumably, vomiting results from stimulation of the area postrema on the floor of the fourth ventricle. Photophobia is another non-specific symptom that occurs in patients with inflammation of the meninges.

Clearly, neurological symptoms due to intracranial disease are confined to the cerebral hemispheres, brainstem, cerbellum and cranial nerves. A principal interconnecting system is the reticular activating system (RAS) which is compromised in many acute neurological emergencies. The integrity of this system is necessary to activate the cerebral cortex and maintain wakefulness. Altered levels of consciousness occur with a bilateral or diffuse anatomical physiological or metabolic disturbance (Plum and Posner, 1980). The impairment involves either the RAS in the upper pons or midbrain or their projections to the thalamus and the cerebral cortex. Because of the potential gravity for serious neurological disability or death, the mildest form of altered arousal demands attention and necessitates an immediate explanation. Depending on the zone and severity of involvement, disorders of the cerebral cortex affect the quality of mental function and are reflected in altered behaviour, poor concentration, flat affect and poor memory, and in inability to calculate, solve problems, recognise patterns or perform complex motor tasks. Abnormalities in language point to an affliction over the lateral portion of the dominant hemisphere. The general practitioner need not know precisely where or why these symptoms are attributed to the encephalon, but only that they are. When the examiner determines that the patient has an altered level of alertness or disordered thinking, further history from a reliable companion or relative should be sought.

With respect to the motor system, several remarks are appropriate concerning intracranial lesions. Disturbances in the motor cortex or its pathways descending through the brainstem result in paralysis or various degrees of weakness, slowness and clumsiness of the contralateral lower face and limbs. Acute structural lesions of the basal ganglia are infrequently manifested by the symptoms of a chronic extra-pyramidal disorder. Rather, compression of the contiguous internal capsule results in a hemiplegia or hemiparesis. Toxic reactions, especially to drugs, sometimes present as spontaneous, involuntary movements, e.g. dystonic contractions of muscles, sudden single (myoclonic) jerks and choreiform movements. Acute lesions of the cerebellum are uncommon and are divided into those involving the hemisphere and the midline or vermis. Acute structural lesions of the cerebellar hemispheres result mostly from infarction. Patients experience dysarthria and poor coordination of the ipsilateral limbs. Conversely, acute lesions of the cerebellar vermis, such as occur with hypertensive haemorrhage, produce a sudden loss in control of the paravertebral muscles and vestibular pathways responsible for an unstable posture and gait. These patients present in a wheelchair or on a stretcher because they are able neither to stand nor to walk, and often are unable to sit up without support. To the unsuspecting examiner, there is a surprising absence of weakness, but, if sought, incoordination of the lower limbs is often present. Thus, in every neurological assessment, an important guideline is to determine whether or not the patient can walk, and if not why not.

Sensory symptoms due to intracranial disease are unlikely features of acute neurological disorders. A reduction or alteration in sensation of the limbs suggests involvement of the contralateral brainstem, thalamus, sensory cortex or their intervening connections. Generally, patients complain of tingling or numbness and, infrequently, pain or loss of thermal sensitivity.

Although isolated cranial nerve lesions occur, it is most important to process the localisation to match acute cranial nerve deficits to long tract motor and sensory deficits that appear with lesions within the brainstem. The cranial nerves subserve both the somatic and accessory respiratory muscles and the primary and special sensory functions of the cranium. The somatic muscles are those of the eyes and tongue, and symptoms include ptosis, double vision, dysarthria and dysphagia. The accessory muscles of respiration are involved in jaw, facial, pharyngeal, laryngeal and head movements. Weakness results in ocular exposure, hoarseness or impaired chewing, sucking, swallowing and head-turning.

Numbness of the face above the eyes and tip of the nose

corresponds to the first division of the trigeminal nerve, over the cheeks and upper lip to the second division, and along the mandible and lower lip to the third division. Disorders of the special senses result in loss of vision, hearing, balance, smell or taste. Acute afflictions of independent cranial nerves are uncommon. Loss of vision is the most serious. Usually the patient complains of blurry and dim vision with compromise of the retina or optic nerve. Homonymous impairment or disturbances such as bright flashes or geometric figures in the visual field imply a structural or physiological alteration in the visual pathways behind the optic chiasm and, usually, in the opposite posterior hemisphere. Because auditory pathways are composed nearly equally of crossed and uncrossed fibres, they are rarely clinically affected by focal neurological deficits. Sudden loss of balance due to a vestibular dysfunction is a frightening experience for many patients. The abrupt sensation of spinning or vertigo is regularly accompanied by nausea or vomiting and aggravated by any change in the position of the head. This disabling situation prompts the patient to think that a stroke is occurring. Disorders of smell and taste are not those of acute neurological disease.

Symptoms below the foramen magnum pertain to the spinal cord, peripheral nervous system and muscle. Recognition of impending spinal cord malfunction, which is not uncommon among patients with metastatic disease, is of critical importance. Vertebral pain results from infection or neoplastic invasion that may eventually compress the spinal cord. Symptoms at the thoracic and lumbar level include weakness and sensory loss of the lower limbs and trunk. With partial lesions, paresis occurs in the ipsilateral extremity, and altered sensation involves the opposite limb. Disturbances of the cervical cord result in additional involvement of the upper extremities. Loss of bladder control or acute retention and distension of the bladder may also occur. Complaints pertaining to the inability to evacuate the bowels or to develop an erection are infrequent.

Acute disorders of the peripheral nerves are characterised by distal motor and sensory complaints. There are several explanations for the distal distribution of these symptoms. Over the trunk of a nerve, there is an accumulative effect on altered conduction due to toxic or inflammatory conditions. Thus, the longer the nerve, the greater the disturbance in conduction and sensory perception. In addition, the small muscles of the distal limbs carry out intricate movements that require patterns of precisely timed discharges. Thus, movement of the smaller, distal muscles is more sensitive to the loss of motor neurones or their axons. Early symptoms of motor dysfunction include stumbling, falling and loss of grip and dexterity. Not infrequently, the paresis encountered in acute neurological emergencies is more profound and results in the inability to walk, stand, or raise the arm. Conversely, the proximal muscles are larger and more actively engaged in tonic contractions that require the expenditure of a large degree of energy to overcome the weight of each limb. Accordingly, diseases of muscle are characterised by proximal weakness. Patients complain about their inability to rise from a chair unassisted, climb stairways, reach overhead shelves or comb their hair. When weakness extends to the paravertebral muscles, patients discover that they are unable to roll over. Sensory disturbances of peripheral nerve disease are also distal. These include numbness and tingling and painful or uncomfortable sensations with stimulation of the affected area. Sharp pain radiating along the course of a peripheral nerve also occurs.

Having assigned the patient's symptoms to areas above or below the foramen magnum and their respective subcompartments, the examiner needs to define the temporal profile of symptoms. This is useful in characterising the underlying pathological process. For example, traumatic and vascular disorders are usually sudden in onset, whereas infections and metabolic and toxic diseases often have a subacute evolution of symptoms. An exact description of where and what the patient was doing at the precise moment of the onset of symptoms is very helpful in defining the abruptness of the neurological event and assisting the patient in recalling any other concurrent symptoms or physiological stresses. Having the patient relate just how the motor, sensory or cognitive malfunction impaired his activity is especially helpful in discerning the magnitude of the symptom.

Additional features in the history assist in estimating the underlying pathology. The occurrence of pain is suggestive of expansion or compression of neural structures or irritation of free nerve endings by inflammation. Episodic symptoms are observed in patients with the neuronal bursts of a seizure or alterations in circulation occurring with vascular disorders. Bilateral and diffuse symptoms are encountered with intoxication and metabolic disturbances of the nervous system.

The history accompanying acute neurological deficits cannot be stressed enough. Frequently, the historical data base constitutes the largest component of an accurate clinical diagnosis. Attention to the foregoing outline should contribute to the clinical method of recognition, localisation and pathological estimation.

## THE EXAMINATION

In acute neurological emergencies, the vital signs are of critical importance. A slow pulse rate in a patient with altered consciousness suggests a dangerously high elevation in intracranial pressure. Altered cardiac rhythms are possibly a telling point in a patient with a focal neurological deficit and cardiogenic embolus. Because of loss of autoregulation of cerebral blood flow with structural lesions of the brain, the need to immediately recognise hypotension in patients with neurological disease cannot be over-emphasised. Perfusion of the focally impaired circulation is directly related to the mean arterial pressure. However, the presence of hypertension in acute neurological disorders requires careful judgement before the blood pressure is lowered. Not infrequently, increased blood pressure is the systematic response to the need for a higher perfusion pressure in patients with intracranial hypertension or with a focal loss in cerebral autoregulation. The alternately slow, shallow and rapid, deep excursions of Cheyne-Stokes respirations clue the clinician to physiological alterations affecting the influence of the cerebral hemispheres on respiration. The bradypnoea is sometimes so profound that it is confused with a respiratory arrest. The sudden appearance of other signs of respiratory release, such as yawning, sighing or hiccuping, are also possible early symptoms of bihemispheric dysfunction. In many instances, the potential for aspiration in comatose patients necessitates intubation and mechanical ventilation. This common procedure obscures observation of the neurogenic influences on patterns of respiration. Thus, the laboured hyperventilation and apneustic breathing associated with upper and lower pontine pathology and the ataxic respirations of medullary lesions are rarely encountered. In addition to documenting fever, the determination of body temperature is necessary to recognise patients with hypothermia associated with thiamin deficiency. hypoadrenalism, hypothyroidism, hypoglycaemia or drug intoxication.

The neurological examination is often conducted in the course of the general physical examination. The purpose is to confirm the location of the neurological disorder suspected by the history. Beginning with the top of the head and ending at the foot, the examination is divided into the mental status and cranial nerves, which are structures located strictly above the foramen magnum, and the motor, reflex and sensory subsystems, which indicate dysfunction either above or below the foramen magnum. If the history regarding motor and sensory function is unremarkable, cerebellar function may be evaluated after the cranial nerves.

In many acute neurological emergencies, the importance of a formal declaration regarding the level of consciousness cannot be overemphasised. Thus, very arbitrary terminology is useful. If other than fully alert, the patient is referred to in the following manner: obtunded, if only a single stimulus arouses the patient to sustained attentiveness; stuporous, if continued stimulation is necessary to maintain the patient's responsiveness to the environment; comatose, if vigorous stimulation fails to elicit a purposeful reaction to the stimulus. Because these terms apply to a fluctuating continuum between wakefulness and coma, the stimulus used and the response elicited should be specifically stated. If consciousness is altered, an extensive examination is limited by the patient's inability to cooperate. Therefore, attention is directed towards determining if the altered level of consciousness is due to impaired activity of the cerebral hemispheres or involves the RAS in the upper brainstem. This achieved by careful observation for signs of brainstem dysfunction reflected in the pupils, eye movements, motor posture and power. These signs also assist in establishing a level of structural or physiological dysfunction in the midbrain, pons or medulla. Consequently, these specific components of the examination are described in detail.

An understanding of pupillary signs is dependent upon a working knowledge of the efferent pathways that influence them. The size of the pupillary aperture is determined by a balance of the parasympathetic and sympathetic nervous system. The parasympathetic influence originates in the Edinger-Westphal nucleus of the rostral midbrain. Pupillomotor fibres pass through the oculomotor nerve, synapse in the ciliary region, and continue as the short ciliary nerves that terminate on the sphincter pupillae muscle. Disruption of these fibres results in mydriasis due to uncontested contraction of the dilator muscle and a fixed reaction to light because of paralysis of the sphincter pupillae. To closely observe the reaction of the iris to light, the 20+ lens of a standard ophthalmoscope is sometimes useful. Impairment of the parasympathetic fibres occurs with compression of the third nerve by the uncus of the temporal lobe, which is forced medially by rapidly evolving hemispheric masses. Often ptosis and adduction paresis from denervation of the levator palpebrae and medial rectus muscle are also present. Bilaterally fixed and dilated pupils are an ominous sign of severe compromise of the rostral midbrain.

9

The sympathetic nervous system originates in the posterior hypothalamus and projects through the reticular formation to the spinal cord, where the pupillomotor fibres exit from the first thoracic segment. There the fibres climb in the sympathetic chain to synapse in the superior cervical ganglion. Post-ganglionic fibres extend around the internal carotid artery and ascend into the cranium. In the cavernous sinus, these axons course with the ophthalmic nerve and travel into the orbit, pass through the ciliary ganglion, and end on the dilator pupillae muscle. Injury to the sympathetic pathway results in miosis from uncontested contraction of the sphincter pupillae muscle and ptosis due to paresis of Mueller's muscle in the upper eyelid. These features of Horner's syndrome are observed in acute neurological emergencies that interrupt the sympathetic pathway in the brainstem, cervical spinal cord or internal carotid artery. Consequently, in these examples of miosis and ptosis there are other severe neurological deficits. In cases of altered consciousness and bilateral miosis, the possibility of bilateral brainstem compression from central-cephalic herniation should be considered. Alternatively, bilateral miosis and impaired consciousness in the absence of other focal neurological deficits occur in patients with metabolic encephalopathies or drug intoxications.

Eye movements are dependent on the integrity of the ocular nerves and their nuclei: the oculomotor nucleus in the rostral midbrain, the trochlear nucleus in the caudal midbrain, and the abducens nucleus in the lower pons. These nuclei receive command signals from the pretectal region for upgaze, the prerubal area for downgaze, and paired zones in the lower, paramedian pons for horizontal gaze. In patients whose impaired consciousness limits voluntary eye movements, vestibulo-ocular reflexes are employed to examine ocular motility. The semicircular canals ordinarily act to maintain the stability of the eyes with respect to gravity by counter-rolling the globes with each movement of the head. Conjugate, lateral eye movements are induced normally by rotating the head in the horizontal plane. A similar oculocephalic manoeuvre in the vertical plane moves the eyes up and down. In head trauma, this manoeuvre should be avoided unless roentgenograms of the cervical vertebrae have excluded a fracture. Caloric stimulation of the semicircular canals by irrigation of the external auditory canals with ice water is a stronger labyrinthine stimulus than oculocephalic rotations. Cold water calorics are used in patients without otitis or discharge from the ear, and are essential in completing the examination if the oculocephalic manoeuvre fails to induce ocular rotations. Tonic, horizontal deviation of the eyes towards the irrigated ear occurs if the vestibulo-ocular pathways from the semicircular canals to the pons and midbrain are intact (Nathanson *et al.*, 1957).

Palsies of the third, fourth or sixth nerves are readily identified by voluntary eye movements or vestibulo-ocular stimulation. Gaze deviations require thoughtful consideration. Downgaze deviation suggests an acute impairment of the pretectal region influencing upgaze which occurs with thalamic haemorrhage or acute hydrocephalus. Upgaze deviation is observed with the rare infarct of the inferior rostral midbrain responsible for downgaze. Bilateral absence of horizontal gaze following oculocephalic manoeuvre and ice water caloric stimulation implicates a severe structural or metabolic impairment of both control centres for horizontal gaze in the lower pons. An indication of drug-induced coma with absent, vestibulo-ocular reflexes is the preservation of pupillary function (Fisher, 1969). Pathological disruption of pontine control for ipsilateral horizontal gaze results in disinhibition of the opposing pons and deviation of the eyes away from the pathological process. The pathologically affected pons is identified by the failure of either oculocephalic rotations or ice water irrigation to induce ipsilateral horizontal gaze. If either of these vestibulo-ocular reflexes overcomes the horizontal gaze deviation and shows a full range of conjugate eye movements, withdrawal of the influence on horizontal gaze by the frontal eye field is implicated. A destructive process in the middle lobule of the frontal lobe or its corticobulbar pathways that decussate in the upper brainstem impairs horizontal gaze directed from the contralateral pons. The disinhibition of the ipsilateral pons results in horizontal gaze deviation towards the affected cerebral hemisphere; this deviation is overcome by vestibular stimulation of the structurally preserved mechanisms for horizontal gaze in the contralateral pons. A hemiparesis from impairment of the nearby corticospinal tract is often present to assist anatomic localisation. Thus, patients with a frontal lobe disorder have a contralateral hemiparesis and ipsilateral deviation of the eyes, and patients with a destructive lesion of the pons have a contralateral hemiparesis and contralateral gaze deviation.

Alterations in the motor system include unilateral or bilateral hemiparesis or hemiplegias if the descending corticospinal tract and related motor pathways are impaired in the cerebral hemisphere, brainstem or spinal cord. In comatose patients, deep pressure on a nailbed is useful to judge the movement of one limb versus the other.

Elicited responses include purposeful or semipurposeful withdrawal, flexion, extension or the absence of movement. More complex posturing includes decorticate or decerebrate movements. In experimental animals, a lesion above the red nucleus in the rostral midbrain or decortication results in a flexor bias of the forelimbs. By analogy, a decorticate posture in man consists of flexion and supination of the forearm and extension of the legs. Decerebration is produced by lesions between the red nucleus and vestibular nucleus in the lower pons and leads to an extensor bias in each limb. A similar decerebrate posture in man is represented by extension and hyperpronation of the forearm with extension of the legs. In the clinical setting pathological processes above and below the red nucleus have pervasive physiological effects that are equivalent to structural lesions. Therefore, decorticate and decerebrate postures are not necessarily caused by destructive lesions even though they are analogous to such lesions in experimental animals. None the less, they are ominous signs of severe compromise of the cerebrum or brainstem.

There are several additional features of the neurological examination that have potential relevance for patients with altered consciousness. The head is inspected for signs of trauma, particularly lacerations, abrasions and ecchymotic areas over the mastoid process (Battle's sign) or around the orbit. Lacerations or contusions of the tongue, lip or inner cheek suggest the possibility of a seizure. Occasionally, fundoscopic examination shows nerve-fibre layer haemorrhages that occur with sudden increases in intracanial pressure. Dot haemorrhages in the retina suggest systematic embolisation or a coagulopathy. Retinal exudates are indicative of systemic diabetes mellitus or hypertension. Because papilloedema results from obstruction in the slow transport of axoplasm in axons forming the optic nerve, it is not surprisingly a sign of subacute or chronically increased intracranial pressure. Papilloedema is infrequently observed in patients with acutely elevated intracanial pressure (Selhorst et al., 1985). The corneal-blink reflex is easily elicited by touching the cornea with a wisp of cotton and observing contraction of each orbicularis oculi. This pontine reflex, however, is variably affected by many acute neurological processes and is not therefore a sensitive indicator of pontine function. However, a related phenomenon is the corneo-mandibular reflex in which stimulation of the cornea is followed by contralateral deviation of the jaw. In one clinical study, this sign occurred in comatose patients with acutely increased intracranial pressure from structural lesions, but not in those patients with coma from metabolic disorders (Guberman, 1982). The gag reflex and medullary drive of respiration are chiefly of value in providing evidence of neurological function in questions of brain death. The Babinski sign or extensor plantar response is useful in confirming the presence of central nervous system disease and, particularly, involvement of the descending corticospinal tract. This sign is elicited by using a noxious stimulus, such as a key, and drawing it along the lateral edge of the foot from the heel and medially across the sole. Normally, all the toes flex in reaction to the stimulus. A typically abnormal response is denoted by extension of the great toe while the remaining toes separate like a fan and flex. Muscle stretch reflexes are often depressed in acute neurological disorders, so they are of minimal value in this setting.

In patients with acute neurological disorders who are alert, the neurological examination is more extensive. To maintain an orderly evaluation, attention is directed first to findings above the foramen magnum. Priority is properly given to cognitive faculties. Comprehension of language is quickly determined by having the patient carry out a few simple motor commands. Slow and dys-arthric speech implicates impairment of the premotor areas of the dominant hemisphere that are programmed for the expression of language. Confusion or impaired immediate memory is suspected when the patient is disoriented to time and place. If these functions are intact, sufficient communication and cooperation enable systematic testing of the cranial nerves subserving vision, eye movements, facial sensation and hearing as well as jaw, facial, pharyngeal and tongue movements. Cerebellar function is examined if the history suggests that pain, weakness or sensory loss would not interfere with testing. The most sensitive overall test is probably the tandem walk. An impaired cerebellar hemisphere is reflected by incoordination of the ipsilateral limbs. This is detected by rapid movements such as repetitively touching the finger to the nose and the examiner's extended finger, alternating pronation and supination of the hand, and rubbing the heel on the shin between the knee and the ankle.

In patients with disease below the foramen magnum, evidence of vertebral disease should be sought by palpation of the spinous processes. Muscle strength is determined by evidence of forceful resistance in each of the principal functional groups of muscles around the major joints, especially the flexors, extensors, abductors and adductors. Muscle tone is easiest to determine by passive

13

movements of the upper extremities. In acute neurological disorders, hypotonicity is common. Subsequently, in patients with lesions of central motor tracts, a spastic increase in tone evolves and passive stretching of the muscles is met by increasing resistance or 'catch' followed by a sudden release of tone. Weakness, spasticity and loss of dexterity result from lesions of the upper motor neurone in the cerebral cortex and its descending pathway through the spinal cord. The lower motor unit refers to the motor neurone in the anterior horn of the spinal cord, its axon travelling in the ventral root and peripheral nerve, and the muscle fibres it innervates. Disease in the lower motor unit results in hypotonicity, loss of muscle bulk and weakness.

In acute neurological disorders muscle stretch reflexes are commonly hypoactive or absent. Within several days these reflexes become hyperactive or clonic and are also a sign of upper motor neurone dysfunction. Because these changes develop over time, the reflex findings are often not useful in acute situations. Furthermore, hypoactive or absent reflexes result from perturbed conduction due to disease of the spinal roots or peripheral nerves. Thus, in acute neurological disorders, hyporeflexia alone will not localise the pathological disturbance.

Sensory disorders are defined by the patterns of denervation with respect to the peripheral nerves, spinal segments or ascending spinal tracts. Central pathways are implicated by homolateral involvement of the trunk and limbs. Sensory loss corresponding to a spinal segment suggests disruption of afferent signals travelling in the dorsal root or in respective segments of the spinal cord. Key segmental landmarks include C-2 at the occiput, C-5 at the shoulder, T-1 at the little finger, T-4 at the nipples, T-10 at the umbilicus, L-1 in the groin, L-5 over the dorsum of the foot, S-1 at the heel, S-3 for the genitalia and S-5 in the perianal region. Sensory loss corresponding to major peripheral nerves includes the shoulder for the axillary nerve, the anatomical snuff box for the radial nerve, the middle finger for the median nerve, the little finger for the ulnar nerve, the anterior thigh for the femoral nerve, the dorsum of the foot for the superficial peroneal nerve, and the sole of the foot for the posterior tibial nerve.

## THE WRITTEN RECORD

The written record is an opportunity to record all meaningful observations made in the course of the history and examination and to reflect upon their implications. The locus and nature of each disturbance affecting the nervous system should be clearly listed in numerical fashion. Confirming neurological signs should be in evidence. A comprehensive diagnostic and management plan is then formulated and appropriately stated.

# REFERENCES

Fisher, C.M. (1969) The neurological examination of the comatose patient. *Acta Neurol. Scand. 45* (Suppl. 36), 1–59

Guberman, A. (1982) Clinical significance of the corneomandibular reflex. *Arch. Neurol. 39*, 578–80

Kurtzke, J.F. (1984) Neuroepidemiology. *Ann. Neurol. 16*, 265–77

Nathanson, M., Bergman, P.S. and Anderson, P.J. (1957) Significance of oculocephalic and caloric responses in the unconscious patient. *Neurology 7*, 829–32

Plum, F. and Posner, J.B. (1980) *The diagnosis of stupor and coma*, F.A. Davis, Philadelphia, 3rd edition, p.4

Selhorst, J.B., Gudeman, S.K., Butterworth, J.F., Harbison, J.W., Miller, J.D. and Becker, D.P. (1985) Papilledema after acute head injury. *Neurosurgery 16*, 357–63

# 2

# Disturbances of Consciousness ('Funny Turns')

Lance D. Blumhardt

## INTRODUCTION

It has been estimated that about 10% of patients presenting to family practitioners will have neurological complaints. Of these, fits, faints and other alterations of consciousness are common. In one study 2.5% of 88 000 patients presented to their family practitioner with either epilepsy or syncope (Stewart, 1976). In another family-practice-based study, epilepsy was the main diagnosis in 12.4% of cases (Murray, 1977). In patients referred to neurological or paediatric clinics, the proportion with some form of disturbed consciousness will be even higher. For example, Tibbles (1976) found that 23% of such referrals had epilepsy and a further 11% were classified on the 'borderlands of epilepsy'.

Recurrent, transient episodes of altered awareness or loss of consciousness may cause considerable alarm in patients and their relatives, particularly at their onset. There are many causes for such symptoms and some are potentially life-threatening. The family practitioner must be competent at recognising the patient whose symptoms justify urgent referral to a cardiologist or neurologist for investigation and treatment.

It has been estimated that 80% of all neurological complaints can be adequately cared for by a properly trained family practitioner (Murray, 1977), but in practice one finds that patients with uncomplicated vaso-vagal syncope are frequently referred to neurological clinics while other cases with typical epileptic seizures are not referred and remain undiagnosed for many years. Judging from the sample of cases that do reach specialist clinics a good deal of diagnostic confusion prevails.

A 45-year-old patient was referred to a neurology clinic with progressive loss of balance. In the course of the interview an additional history emerged of attacks characterised by a dreamy feeling, *déjà vu* and occasional falls. These were occurring weekly and had been present for 35 years! The patient, who drove a car, had been told by several doctors that the symptoms 'could not remotely be epilepsy' although the patient had suggested this diagnosis (correctly) herself. Following intensive investigations the neurologist was unable to explain the cause of the cerebellar ataxia but the temporal lobe seizures ceased immediately with the introduction of carbamazepine.

Although at first sight the diagnostic possibilities for recurrent transient episodes of disturbed consciousness appear to be multitudinous (Table 2.1), common things occur commonly. Most cases coming to family practitioners will turn out to have either epilepsy or syncope. Although there is a considerable overlap in the symptomatology of faints and fits, there are a few key features which, if assembled in the correct sequence, will reliably distinguish these conditions in the majority of cases.

It is reasonable to begin by deciding whether the evidence is sufficient to sustain a diagnosis of epilepsy. The history must be taken in great detail, prompting the patient to keep the account in sequence and probing for the earliest warning symptoms as well as the events leading up to the attack. If a diagnosis of epilepsy cannot be made, then common causes of syncope should be considered depending on the *circumstances* of the attacks and other clues.

## IS IT A FORM OF EPILEPSY?

Despite a widely prevalent faith in high-technology medicine and a firm belief that 'tests' can provide the answer, the diagnosis of epilepsy remains primarily a question of applying clinical skills in history taking. A complete diagnosis of epilepsy requires three conditions to be satisfied; first, the symptoms must be recognised to be epilepsy; secondly, the type of epilepsy must be defined; and, finally, the cause of the seizures needs to be established. This account will be concerned primarily with the first two parts of the diagnosis for which it is necessary to know a few facts about the different types of epilepsy.

*Major convulsions* usually present few diagnostic difficulties

17

**Table 2.1:** Causes of episodic disturbance of consciousness or altered awareness

| | |
|---|---|
| **Epilepsy** | Grand mal ('tonic/clonic', major)<br>Temporal lobe ('complex partial seizures')<br>Simple focal (motor or sensory)<br>Petit mal<br>Minor |
| **Syncope** | Vaso-vagal (simple faints)<br>Cardiac<br>   arrhythmias<br>   outflow obstruction<br>Micturition syncope<br>Cough syncope<br>Carotid sinus syncope<br>Reflex ('vagal') anoxic seizures<br>Postural hypotension |
| **Basilar ischaemia** | Migraine<br>Thromboembolic (vertebro-basilar transient ischaemic attack)<br>Mechanical (spondylotic) compression of vertebral arteries |
| **Drop attacks** | Cryptogenic, of middle-aged women |
| **Psychiatric** | Hyperventilation attacks<br>Pseudoseizures ('hysterical attacks') |
| **Metabolic** | Hyperglycaemia<br>Hypocalcaemia |
| **Miscellaneous** | Transient global amnesia<br>Severe vertigo (Ménière's disease)<br>Breath-holding attacks in infancy<br>Intermittent obstructive hydrocephalus<br>Narcolepsy/cataplexy<br>Unrecognised trauma |

Source: Adapted with permission from Blumhardt (1986)

unless they were single or unwitnessed incidents. The relevance of the tonic spasm, rhythmic clonic movements, tongue-biting, incontinence, respiratory changes and cyanosis need hardly be emphasised. The patient and the eye witness should be questioned closely for any sequelae such as injuries, confusion, retrograde amnesia or tiredness. Although recurrent disturbances of sleep such as odd noises, falling out of bed, nocturnal incontinence or confusion may be non-specific in themselves, they often provide suggestive clues to the diagnosis of epilepsy in young adults.

The patient must be closely questioned for the *earliest* warnings of his attacks as these may provide characteristic evidence of epilepsy, as well as clues to the likely site of the epileptic focus (e.g. the rising epigastric sensation of a temporal lobe seizure or the forced turning of head or eyes to one side in a frontal discharge). The eye witness should be questioned to establish the presence of rigidity or tonic spasm. Was the patient limp or floppy, or stiff and rigid? Was the jaw slack or clamped? The essential rhythmic nature of tonic–clonic movements or myoclonic jerking should be distinguished from the tremulousness or shaking associated with fright or emotion.

The circumstances of the attack should be established, as convulsions may occur in some patients only under specific provocation, for example during alcohol withdrawal, after certain drugs (e.g. phenothiazines or tricyclics) or as a secondary complication of a faint. If the circumstances are consistent with a faint, but a seizure is suggested by the history, the position of the patient at the time of the event should be established. Was he held up or propped against a wall causing further anoxia? If so the seizure was probably due to secondary anoxia and the patient should not be regarded as epileptic. All too often the failure to recognise the circumstances of the attacks leads to erroneous conclusions and mismanagement.

Brief attacks of loss of consciousness or unresponsiveness occurring for the first time in adult life are likely to be *temporal lobe epilepsy* (TLE), now known as complex partial seizures (CPS), but such patients are frequently misdiagnosed as 'petit mal'. Scarcely a month goes by without the receipt of a referral letter illustrating this area of confusion.

> This 60-year-old man has recently developed petit mal. His blank spells in which he is unresponsive for one or two minutes are occurring several times a week and appear to be followed by a little confusion. They are not responding to ethosuximide. Could you please advise?

If the attacks began in adult life, if the duration of unresponsiveness is more than 20 seconds, if falling and incontinence are involved, if there is a warning ('aura') and if there are sequelae such as injury or confusion, it is *not* petit mal epilepsy (Table 2.2).

The diagnosis of CPS (TLE) should be immediately suggested if the patient describes the characteristic warnings of an odd sensation starting in the epigastrium and rising into the chest or towards the head. This autonomic aura is much more common than the widely recognised olfactory and gustatory hallucination emphasised by

19

**Table 2.2:** Some features distinguishing temporal lobe from petit mal epilepsy

|  | Temporal lobe epilepsy | Petit mal epilepsy |
|---|---|---|
| **Onset** | Any age | Childhood |
| **Aura** | Epigastric sensation, *déjà vu*, olfactory, gustatory, vertigo, etc. | Nil |
| **'Absence'** | Usually 2 to 3 minutes | < 20 seconds (usually < 10 seconds) |
| **Movements** | Common (automatisms) swallowing; lip-smacking; chewing; fumbling with hands; walking aimlessly; falls | Uncommon: occasional twitch; flickering eyelids; rare falls |
| **Autonomic features** | Common: flushing/pallor; tachycardia/bradycardia; sweating; apnoea | Rare: may be slight flushing/pallor |
| **Sequelae** | Common: amnesia; confusion | Nil |

Source: Adapted with permission from Blumhardt (1986).

textbooks. It is often associated with a dreamy detached feeling, an intense sensation of familiarity (*déjà vu*) or distortions of temporal and spatial awareness. The eye witness will generally be able to recall the blank, glassy stare, colour changes (pallor *or* flushing) and any repetitive semi-complex automatic movements such as lip-smacking, chewing, swallowing or, for example, clenching and unclenching of the fists (automatisms). Occasionally, attacks may be characterised by strange and inappropriate behaviour which may persist for long periods (complex partial status, psychomotor status), but the duration of most temporal-lobe seizures is a matter of several minutes. The distinction from the childhood absence attack (petit mal) is important because the medication required is different and because temporal lobe seizures are *focal* seizures which may require further investigation to exclude underlying structural lesions. It is often difficult to obtain a conclusive history due to the reservations that many patients have in describing what may seem to them to be ludicrous, embarrassing or indescribable symptoms. One must not accept a patient's vague initial story but should make repeated attempts and prompts to build up a fuller and more accurate account of the sequence of events. An understanding and sympathetic manner is essential, and it is often necessary to ask the patient directly about each of the odd feelings to establish their nature.

Petit mal epilepsy is an uncommon problem in adult neurology. It is a precisely defined clinical entity requiring a characteristic EEG abnormality of regular spike and slow-wave activity at a frequency of exactly 3 per second. Although it may persist into early adult life, the onset must be in *childhood*. It *very rarely* starts after the age of 15 years. A sudden arrest of speech or activity (often recognised for the first time during reading) with loss of attention or 'absence' for a few seconds (of which the patient is usually unaware), is characteristic. The longest attacks are 20 seconds but most are shorter. There may be circumoral pallor, slight flushing, flickering of the eyes or even a twitch of the limbs, but usually there are no movements or other signs at all and the brief periods of unresponsiveness may go unrecognised by all but the most alert parent or teacher.

Another common diagnostic error is to confuse transient ischaemic attacks (TIA, which rarely involve disturbed consciousness) with focal motor seizures (these epileptic patients not infrequently arrive in my clinic taking aspirin!). This distinction should not be difficult if it is remembered that epilepsy is largely a 'positive' phenomenon (i.e. the superimposition of unwanted rhythmic motor activity), whereas TIAs are characterised in the main by 'negative' features (i.e. loss of function or normal sensation causing paralysis or numbness).

If the characteristic features of the different types of epilepsy are not evident after a detailed interrogation of the patient and the eye witness, other causes of blackouts should be considered (Table 2.1). It is essential to have an understanding of syncope in its various forms as this is the next most likely diagnosis after epilepsy and is usually easily distinguishable (Table 2.3).

## IS IT SOME SORT OF FAINT?

Here the key to the diagnosis lies in the *history of the* circumstances *of each attack. It is extraordinary how often* patients who faint in entirely appropriate circumstances are misdiagnosed as epileptic. One can only assume that the golden question, 'What were you doing at the time?', is seldom asked. The eye-witness account is often crucial.

In the majority of healthy non-pregnant patients prolonged

**Table 2.3:** Some features helpful in distinguishing epilepsy from syncope

|  | Epilepsy | Syncope |
| --- | --- | --- |
| **Circumstances** | Any posture, onset in sleep/morning common | Prolonged standing; sudden postural change |
| **Warning** | Aura rising epigastric sensation in TLE *déjà vu*<br><br>Focal motor/sensory symptoms | Pre-syncope tinnitus; light-headedness; blurring vision; sweating (clamminess); warmth; nausea |
| **Collapse/loss of consciousness** | Sudden +/− cry/scream; rigid/stiff; bitten tongue/lip or cheek; rhythmic jerks<br><br>Injuries common | Gradual 'slump'; limp; floppy; still ('dead'); occasional twitch; fluttering eyelids<br><br>Injuries uncommon |
| **Colour** | Blue/grey pale | Waxy pale |
| **Incontinence** | Common | Uncommon (can occur with full bladder) |
| **Recovery** | Slow (minutes/days); confused/amnesic; abnormal speech/ behaviour; drowsy; sleep; muscle pain; malaise; lethargy | Rapid (seconds to minutes) |

Source: Adapted with permission from Blumhardt (1986).

standing or sudden postural change is necessary for a faint. Other provoking circumstances may be obvious, for example a crowded stuffy room, a painful injection or rectal examination or sudden emotion (*vaso-vagal syncope*). Usually patients are aware of feeling light-headed with blurred vision, muffling of sounds, sweatiness and warmth ('pre-syncope') and the faint may be averted by lying down. Eye witnesses are likely to be able to confirm the circumstances, the slump to the floor, the limpness of the limbs, the sweating, the lack of clonic movements or rigidity and the profound and 'waxy' pallor which persists for a surprisingly long time after the faint. Although vaso-vagal syncope can *recur* in later life, it should not be diagnosed in adults who do not have a history of fainting in adolescence. When there are no obvious predisposing causes, the patient should be carefully assessed to exclude other factors such as anaemia, cardiac disease and postural hypotension. This is particularly important in the middle-aged and elderly.

Young men who 'collapse' in the bathroom or on the way back to bed in the early hours of the morning are in considerable danger of being treated with anticonvulsants and losing their driving licence. The circumstances alone should suggest *micturition syncope*, but the delusion that this condition is limited to elderly men with prostatism seems widespread. It can occur at any age, but the typical victim is healthy and in his third or fourth decade (Eberhart and Morgan, 1960). Even if a secondary seizure results from anoxia (this may happen if the patient is propped or held up in the faint, e.g., against the bath in a small bathroom or held up by the spouse), such patients must not be diagnosed as epileptic.

Another group of patients who cause great alarm in parents and family practitioners and are likely to receive an inappropriate prescription for anticonvulsants (in one series as many as 40% had been so treated) are children whose faints are triggered by minor trauma and complicated by rigidity, pallor, a few twitches and sometimes incontinence (*non*-epileptic reflex 'vagal' anoxic seizures) (Stephenson, 1978). These episodes often cause panic when they occur in the out-patient clinic during venepuncture or in the playground, when they follow a relatively trivial but painful knock. The drama of the secondary anoxic seizure often misleads the GP although the history of the precipitating factors is usually obvious enough if pursued. The mechanism of the attacks is an exaggerated reflex vagal bradycardia or asystole caused by the painful stimulus. If treatment is required for frequent attacks, it is with long-acting atropine derivatives and *not* anticonvulsants.

The crucial importance of the eye witness is emphasised by faints that occur in the context of violent coughing bouts (*cough syncope*) (Sharpey-Schafer, 1953). These patients typically suffer from chronic airways disease and lack insight into the severity of their coughing and its relationship to their blackouts. They often appear to be 'amnesic' for the bout of coughing that precipitates their blackout. Thus the cause of their syncope may only be established via an eye witness.

When middle-aged or elderly patients present with syncopal episodes precipitated by head-turning or perhaps a tight collar, the rare condition of *carotid sinus syncope* should be considered (Hutchinson and Stock, 1960). The heightened sensitivity of the baroreceptor mechanism is thought to be due to atheroma in the wall of the carotid sinus. In these cases profound bradycardia or asystole may result from the slightest pressure on the neck. It is important to distinguish this condition from epilepsy as surgical treatment may relieve the symptoms.

Diagnostic confusion may arise when a faint with a full bladder results in incontinence. Epilepsy is unlikely in the absence of stiffness, clonic jerking, tongue-biting, or 'post-ictal' confusion. However, when a patient faints into a sitting position (e.g. propped against the bath in a small bathroom as may occur in micturition syncope), the secondary deep cerebral anoxia may precipitate a tonic seizure with rigidity and incontinence or even a full-blown convulsion. This situation ('complicated syncope') can be solved by a detailed history of the predisposing circumstances, the sequence of events, and an eyewitness account of the position in which the fit occurred. When rigidity and twitching occur in such cases, there is usually a rapid recovery with none of the usual sequelae of the epileptic seizure.

In a patient suffering from heart disease and palpitations, syncopal attacks could well be due to life-threatening cardiac arrhythmias such as heart block (*Stokes–Adams syndrome*) although this is an uncommon cause of loss of consciousness compared with epilepsy. A slow or markedly irregular pulse in such patients is an indication for ECG studies and rapid referral to a cardiologist.


## IS IT SOMETHING ELSE?

The majority of funny turns will turn out to be either fits or faints. However, other uncommon or rare causes of altered awareness as listed in Table 2.1 must be considered in particular circumstances.

Although some patients with *migraine* may sink into a semi-coma during their headaches (Bickerstaff, 1961), the onset is slow, they can be roused temporarily from their stupor, and an associated headache and vomiting usually indicate the reason for their drowsiness.

*Basilar ischaemia* as a cause of *repeated* transient episodes of loss of consciousness, whether by mechanical interference with vertebral artery flow by cervical spondylotic disease or by microemboli, is much overdiagnosed, generally on dubious grounds. Most neurologists would find it very difficult to think of even a single case with whom to convince their colleagues. The diagnosis should only be entertained when obvious evidence of vertebro-basilar ischaemia such as diplopia, vertigo, alternating hemiplegia or circumoral paraesthesiae is associated with the attacks.

There are many causes of unexplained falls or *drop attacks* but

**Table 2.4:** Some proposed causes of falls or 'drop attacks'

| Aetiology | Reference |
|---|---|
| Benign cryptogenic of females | Stevens and Matthews, 1973 |
| Epilepsy | Lennox and Lennox, 1960 |
| Cervical spondylosis | Sheehan et al., 1960 |
| Vertebro-basilar insufficiency | Williams and Wilson, 1962 |
| Progressive supranuclear palsy | Steele et al., 1964 |
| Congenital heart disease | Evans and Bremner, 1961 |
| Colloid cyst of third ventricle | Kelly, 1951 |
| Foramen magnum tumours | Kremer, 1958 |
| Myxoedema | Jellinek, 1962 |
| Old age | Sheldon, 1960 |
| Menopausal muscular dystrophy | Shy and McEachern, 1951 |
| Subconscious guilt (erotic thought) | Leuba, 1950 |

some of these are notoriously difficult to verify (Table 2.4). One should always determine whether there is loss of consciousness as patients with weakness of the quadriceps may have sudden catastrophic falls and I have seen patients with myasthenia gravis extensively investigated for 'blackouts'. A history will readily exclude syncope and cataplexy as possible causes of sudden falls.

A particularly characteristic presentation is the middle-aged female who has sudden inexplicable falls when shopping (*cryptogenic drop attacks*). There is no obvious loss of consciousness but the fall may cause injuries to hands, knees or face. The cause of these distressing attacks remains unknown. Provided the history is typical and there are no abnormal signs, investigations are unnecessary as these episodes are benign and tend to remit spontaneously (Stephens and Matthews, 1973).

Other episodic symptoms may have a *psychiatric* basis. Attacks in the anxious patient which are characterised by hyperventilation, tetany and circumoral or peripheral tingling are usually easy enough to diagnose (*hyperventilation syndrome*), but malingerers or hysterical patients with seizure-like episodes may require in-patient observation and monitoring to differentiate genuine epilepsy from *'pseudoseizures'* or hysterical attacks. (Roy, 1979).

*Hypoglycaemia* must always be kept in mind when patients complain of transient confusion, disturbed behaviour, fear, sweating and other neurological and sympathetic symptoms. A blood glucose should always be taken if a patient is seen during an undiagnosed attack.

Middle-aged patients occasionally present with a history of

transient loss of memory. The event is usually single and the gap in memory short (minutes or hours) and permanent. During the episode the patient may be agitated, asking repeated questions, although orientation in self is often preserved (*transient* global amnesia). *It should be distinguished from temporal lobe epilepsy.*

The underlying problem is usually obvious enough in the rare patient with *Ménière's disease* in whom a transient blackout may occur during a violent attack of vertigo.

Infants up to the age of 3 years who become upset and cry may suddenly stop breathing and appear to be unconscious, stiff and blue (*breath-holding attacks*). These attacks can be distinguished from epilepsy by the history of the provoking event which upset or frustrated the child.

Patients with *obstructive hydrocephalus* usually have headaches and neurological signs including papilloedema. Sufferers from *narcolepsy* will be able to distinguish the inappropriate sleep and falls due to *cataplexy* from episodes of loss of consciousness.

## CONCLUSIONS

If each case is regarded as a diagnostic challenge, the practitioner will find that, more often than not, surprisingly little 'detective' work is required to reach a preliminary diagnosis. The GP is in an ideal position to obtain critical diagnostic information from patients and relatives before memories have faded. He should then have a sound basis for deciding whether the patient should be sent to a neurologist or a cardiologist.

Where the diagnosis remains problematic it is most often due to an inadequate history of events. This may be because the circumstances or the aura are confounded by amnesia, because the patient cannot describe his unusual experiences or because no eye witness is available. In many cases it is helpful to re-take and check the history. Many patients referred to neurology clinics with 'unexplained' attacks are diagnosed on the history alone. Contrary to popular belief the diagnosis or the prognosis can seldom be provided by the EEG. Epilepsy, in the great majority of cases, remains a clinical diagnosis. When doubt persists despite a full neurological assessment, *it is far better to delay* a diagnosis in an epileptic than to diagnose epilepsy in error. The temptation of 'therapeutic trials' with anticonvulsants should be resisted as they frequently cause further confusion and complicate future management. It is wiser in most situations to procrastinate until the passage of time and further events provide the conclusive information.

## NOTE

Portions of the text have been adapted with permission from Blumhardt (1986).

## REFERENCES

Bickerstaff, E.R. (1961) Basilar migraine. *Lancet 1*, 15

Blumhardt, L.D. (1986) Fits, faints and funny turns. *The Practitioner 230*, 117

Eberhart, C. and Morgan, J.W. (1960) Micturition syncope. *J. Amer. Med. Assn 174*, 2076

Evans, D.W. and Bremner, O. (1961) Drop attacks in cyanotic congenital heart disease. *Lancet 2*, 575

Hutchinson, E.C. and Stock, J.P. (1960) The carotid sinus syndrome. *Lancet 2*, 445

Jellinek, E.H. (1962) Fits, faints, coma and dementia in myxoedema. *Lancet 2*, 1010

Kelly, R. (1951) Colloid cysts of the third ventricle. *Brain 74*, 23

Kremer, M. (1958) Sitting, standing and walking. *Brit. Med. J. ii*, 63

Lennox, W.G. and Lennox, M.A. (1960) *Epilepsy and related disorders* Churchill, London, p. 144

Leuba, T. (1950) Women who fall. *Int. J. Psychoanalysis 31*, 6

Murray, T.J. (1977) Relevance in undergraduate neurological teaching. *Le Journal Canadien des Sciences Neurologiques 4*, 131

Roy, A. (1979) Hysterical seizures. *Arch. Neurol. 36*, 447

Sharpey-Schafer, E.P. (1953) The mechanism of syncope after coughing. *Brit. Med. J. 2*, 860

Sheehan, S., Bauer, R.B. and Meyer, J.S. (1960) Vertebral artery compression in cervical spondylosis: arteriographic demonstration during life of vertebral artery insufficiency due to rotation and extension of the neck. *Neurology 10*, 968.

Sheldon, J.H. (1960) On natural history of falls in old age. *Brit. Med. J. ii*, 1685

Shy, G.M. and McEachern, D. (1951) The clinical features and response to cortisone of menopausal muscular dystrophy. *J. Neurol. Neurosurg. Psychiat. 14*, 101

Steele, J.C., Richardson, J.C. and Olszewski, J. (1964) Progressive supranulcear palsy. *Arch. Neurol. (Chic.) 10*, 333

Stephens, D.D. and Matthews, W.B. (1973) Cryptogenic drop attacks: an affliction of woman. *Brit. Med. J. i*, 439-42

Stephenson, J.P.B. (1978) Reflex anoxic seizures ('white breath-holding'): non-epileptic vagal attacks. *Arch. Dis. Child. 43*, 193

Stewart, W. (1976) Clinical implications of the Virginia study. *J. Family Practice 3*, 10

Tibbles, J.A.R. (1976) The functions and the training of a pediatric neurologist. *Devel. Med. Child Neurol. 18*, 167

Williams, D. and Wilson, T.G. (1962) Diagnosis of major and minor syndromes of basilar insufficiency. *Brain 85*, 741

# 3

# Head Injury

A. David Mendelow

Head injuries are badly managed in accident and emergency
departments and neurosurgeons are partly to blame.

Teasdale (1984)

## INTRODUCTION

This criticism stems from the problem created by the multitude of
head-injured patients that far exceed the small number of beds
available in neurosurgical centres. The majority must be managed in
non-specialised centres often staffed by the inexperienced who are
on duty during the anti-social hours when these patients present to
hospital. In the United Kingdom, for example, one million head-
injured patients attend hospital each year, but there are only about
100 accredited neurosurgeons: approximately 10000 potential head-
injured patients for each neurosurgeon per year! The problem is
compounded by the fact that neurosurgeons prefer to avoid filling
their few beds with the 150000 patients actually admitted to hospital
each year. There are no figures for the total number of beds under
the care of neurosurgeons in the United Kingdom, but probably a
figure of 2500 would be close and only about 500 of these
neurosurgical beds are occupied by people with head injuries. The
vast majority of these patients are therefore cared for by non-
neurosurgeons. The way they are managed and who manages them
differ enormously from place to place. Similarly, the enthusiasm for
caring for these 'unwanted' patients in general, orthopaedic, and
other wards varies. Fortunately, most are mild injuries and two-
thirds are discharged from hospital within 48 hours. However, the
danger is that a few of these mild injuries will develop serious and

life-threatening complications, which need urgent referral to a neurosurgical centre. Delay in the transfer of patients with traumatic intracranial haematomas will result in increased morbidity and mortality.

The problem, therefore, is to find the best management strategy for the wide spectrum of different hospitals and clinics. To standardise treatment, a group of neurosurgeons, orthopaedic surgeons, general surgeons, accident and emergency (A&E) specialists and radiologists have drawn up guidelines which have been published in the *British Medical Journal* ('A Group of Neurosurgeons', 1984) and have now been adopted widely in the United Kingdom. These guidelines indicate:

(1) which patients require a skull X-ray;
(2) who should be admitted to hospital; and
(3) who should be referred to a neurosurgical department.

These guidelines are set out in the Appendix, and will be referred to frequently in this chapter. They are based upon the results of studies of large numbers of head-injured patients in Glasgow and elsewhere. These studies have singled out those patients who are at risk of developing serious complications. The risks are based on a few selected features which are rapid and cheap to ascertain. Because CT scanning is *not* available in the majority of hospitals in the United Kingdom and in many other countries, other factors have to be used to sort these patients into high- and low-risk categories. There will always be hospitals where it is not possible or practical to send every head-injured patient for a CT scan. In these circumstances, reference to the guidelines given at the end of this chapter should be useful.

## PATHOPHYSIOLOGY OF HEAD INJURY

There are different classifications of head injury, but the most useful is the division of brain damage into *primary* and *secondary* types (Table 3.1). *Primary*, or impact, damage occurs at the time of the injury, and is usually unresponsive to treatment. By contrast, *secondary* brain damage occurs *after* the initial impact, is amenable to treatment and can be prevented. This classification is practical and is preferred to the purer pathological division into focal and diffuse brain damage. Initial assessment soon after the injury will indicate

**Table 3.1:** Pathological classification of traumatic brain damage

*Primary brain damage*
1. Diffuse axonal injury
2. Contusions and lacerations of the cortex
3. Primary vascular lesions

*Secondary brain damage*
Extracranial
 1. Hypoxia
 2. Hypotension
Intracranial
 1. Acute traumatic intracranial haematoma: extradural; subdural; intracerebral
 2. Infection: meningitis; brain abscess
 3. Brain swelling: oedema; vascular engorgement
Consequences of complications
 1. Raised intracranial pressure
 2. Intracranial shift and herniation
 3. Cerebral ischaemia

the severity of the primary damage. The patient's subsequent clinical course indicates whether or not secondary brain damage is occurring. This is the basis for the time-honoured but dated principle which dictates that head-injured patients should be observed, and if deterioration takes place, then and only then should they be referred. Implicit in this obsolete dogma is the acceptance that only patients with established brain damage are sent for treatment. Ideally, patients at risk of developing secondary brain damage should be identified *before* deterioration (secondary brain damage) takes place. The identification of risk factors for haematomas (Mendelow *et al.*, 1983) has led to agreement on guidelines for the management of head injury and should reduce secondary brain damage by ensuring that treatment is instituted at the earliest possible stage. Nevertheless in any head injury, if deterioration *does* take place, then it is clear that secondary brain damage is occurring and urgent treatment is called for.

**Primary brain damage**

Primary brain damage is divided into focal and diffuse types.

### Focal brain damage

Contusions and lacerations of the brain are easily recognised macroscopically. They produce their clinical effects by disrupting cortical structures and white matter connections.

### Diffuse brain damage

Diffuse axonal injury (DAI) is now recognised as a common disorder in severe head injury. In patients with DAI, shearing injuries of white matter results in disruption of axons with axonal retraction balls and subsequent formation of microglial stars (Figure 3.1). The white matter lesions may be extensive and may manifest as disruption of the corpus callosum (Figure 3.2). DAI has now been produced experimentally, particularly with angular acceleration injury, and has also been recognised as a cause of the more severe concussional states. Primary *ischaemic* damage may also occur when the initial insult is so severe as to cause apnoea with hypoxia or hypotension and decreased cerebral perfusion pressure (CPP).

## Secondary brain damage

Secondary brain damage may occur as a result of *extracranial* insults such as hypoxia or hypotension. This type of *secondary hypoxia* may be due to airway obstruction, associated chest injury or other pulmonary complications. *Hypotension* is most often due to haemorrhagic shock from multiple injuries. An associated spinal cord injury may also produce both hypoxia and hypotension. These extracranial injuries are common and they adversely affect the outcome (Table 3.2).

The *intracranial* complications that produce secondary brain damage are haemorrhage, brain swelling and infection.

### Haemorrhage

Haemorrhage is frequently localised in the form of a haematoma which may be extradural or intradural.

*Extradural haematomas.* Extradural haematomas are common as part of a skull injury where there may be surprisingly little primary brain damage. The bleeding into the extradural space causes secondary compression of the hemisphere with elevated intracranial pressure (ICP) and subsequent neurological deterioration often from an initially relatively conscious state. Of course, an extradural

**Figure 3.1:** Axonal retraction balls seen with diffuse damage to white matter 6 days after injury. (Palmgren × 250. From Adams, J.H. *et al.* (1977) *Brain* **100**, 489–502, with permission.)

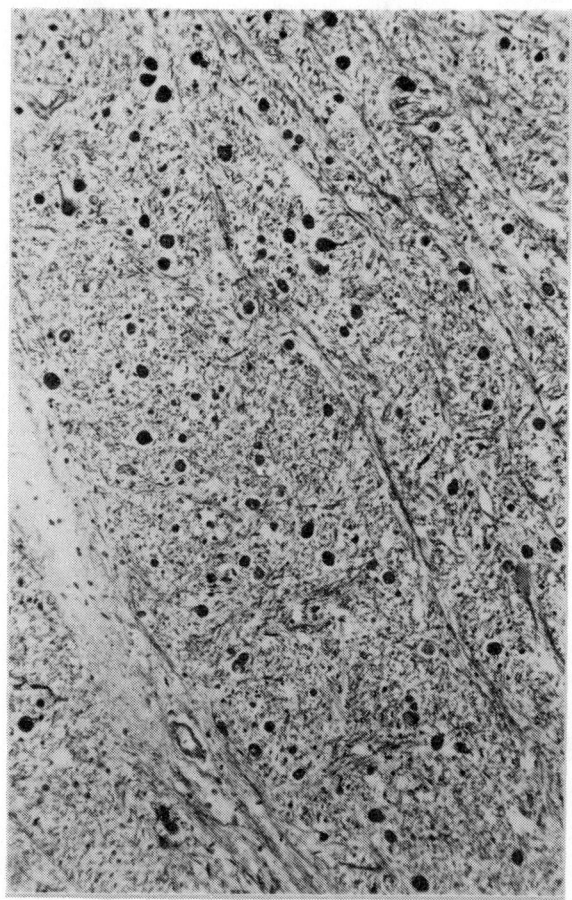

haematoma may occur in a patient with severe brain damage as well, and in that case deterioration may occur from a state of disturbed consciousness *ab initio*.

*Intradural haematomas.* Intradural haematomas were formerly often separated into subdural and intracerebral haematomas. CT scanning has revealed that these two types of haematoma often coexist so that they are better regarded together as intradural. They are usually associated with severe primary brain damage which is why the

33

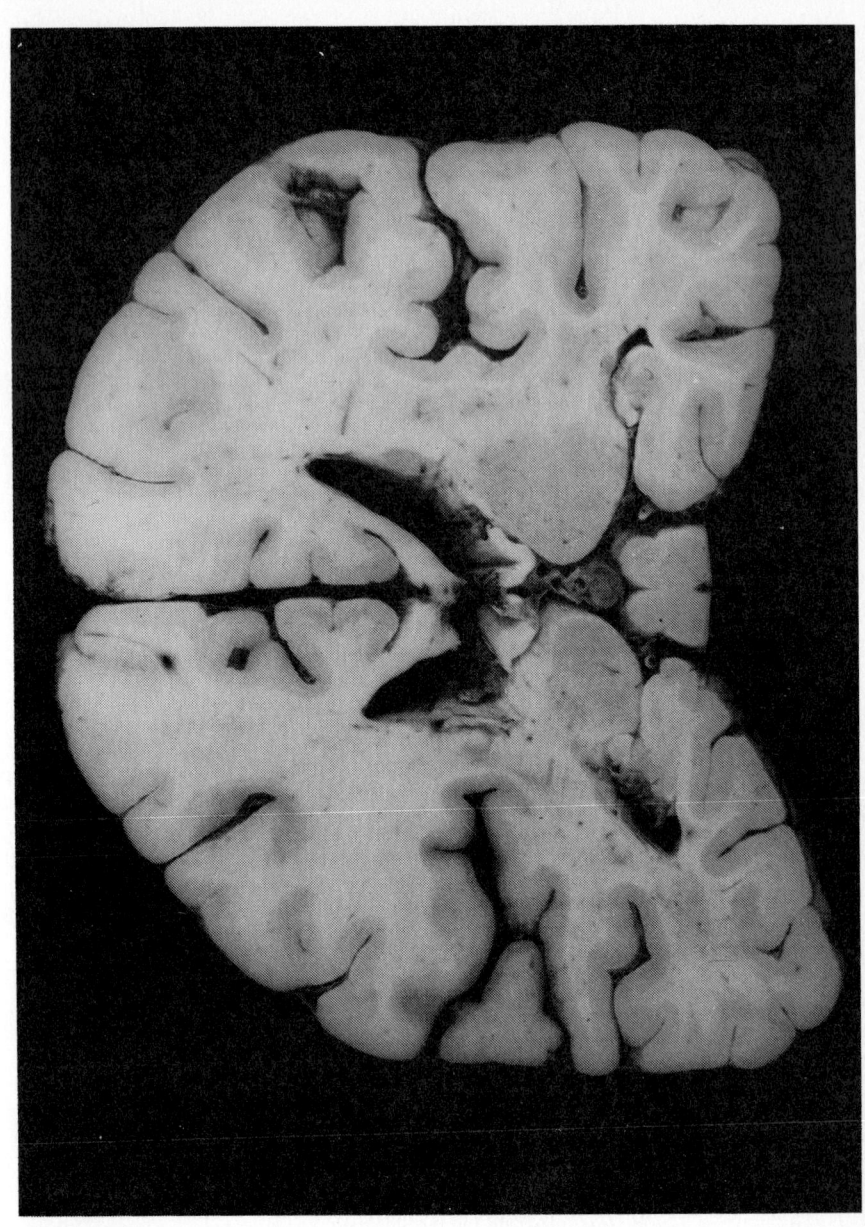

**Figure 3.2:** Coronal section of brain showing disruption of the corpus callosum as part of a diffuse axonal injury

**Table 3.2:** Extracranial insults and outcome. Effect of presence or absence of extracranial insults on outcome from severe head injury

| | Poor outcome (%) in patients with and without extracranial insults | | |
| | Kohi *et al.* (1984) | Gentleman and Jennett (1981) | Miller and Becker (1982) |
| --- | --- | --- | --- |
| Hypoxia and hypotension | 100 | 100 | |
| Hypotension alone | 88 | 75 | 65 |
| Hypoxia alone | 71 | 59 | 65 |
| Neither insult | 27 | 34 | 36 |

Poor outcome = dead, vegetative or severely disabled

mortality is much higher than with the extradural haematoma. Unfortunately, intradural haematomas are more common than extradural haematomas.

*Brain swelling*

Brain swelling may occur as a result of venous engorgement, or may be due to brain oedema. Oedema may be *vasogenic* with damage to the blood–brain barrier and extravasation of the protein from capillaries into the interstitial space. *Cytotoxic* oedema occurs with ischaemia and hypoxia causing damage to the cells, which undergo swelling. *Interstitial* oedema is seen with hydrocephalus where cerebrospinal fluid (CSF) under pressure passes from the ventricle into the subependymal white matter.

*Infection*

Infection usually causes secondary brain damage several days after the injury. Any breach of the dura allows bacteria to contaminate the brain and the CSF pathways. Meningitis is especially common after CSF rhinorrhoea or otorrhoea. It may occur with any basal fracture even in the absence of an overt leak. Brain abscess may be caused by indriven contaminated material, especially with a compound depressed fracture.

## INITIAL MANAGEMENT IN THE CASUALTY DEPARTMENT

The goal in managing patients with head injury must be to prevent secondary brain damage, and initial and secondary extracranial factors must be detected and treated. There is evidence that patients continue to be transferred to neurosurgical units without adequate resuscitation, and it is essential that these correctable causes of brain damage are treated and that patients are stabilised *before* transfer. Their correction is sometimes accompanied by rapid recovery of consciousness, and if treatment is sufficiently prompt it then becomes apparent that there is very little primary brain damage.

The first priority, therefore, is to ensure an adequate airway. Not only should this be patent but adequate gas exchange should be ensured. If there is any respiratory difficulty or cyanosis, the larynx should be inspected with a laryngoscope. If the patient tolerates the insertion of the laryngoscope without gagging, an endotracheal tube should be inserted and, if necessary, ventilation should be initiated. Arterial blood gas analysis should always be performed, and if there is hypoxia despite oxygen therapy ($P_aO_2$ < 60 mmHg) or hypercapnia ($P_aCO_2$ > 45 mmHg), then intubation and ventilation is necessary. If the patient is struggling, great care should be taken to avoid aggravating the situation and an anaesthetist may be required to administer drugs to assist intubation. Here again, care should be taken to avoid periods of apnoea or underventilating the patient. If the patient has hypoxia or hypercapnia, despite spontaneous hyperventilation clinically before intubation, then it is particularly important that the patient should be hyperventilated because failure to do so will result in further deterioration in the arterial blood gases. This is sometimes seen if a normal minute volume is prescribed in a patient who was hyperventilating spontaneously before intubation. In other words, blood gases should be checked soon after intubation to ensure a low or normal $P_aCO_2$.

Simultaneously, the pulse and blood pressure should be measured and an intravenous infusion commenced. If the pulse rate is greater than 120 per minute, or if the systolic blood pressure is less than 100 mmHg, colloid should be infused immediately and when possible a central venous pressure (CVP) line should be inserted. In the absence of hypotension, normal intravenous fluid volumes should be administered. It goes without saying that external haemorrhage should be stopped. In its absence, and if there is hypotension, internal haemorrhage should be suspected and investigated appropriately with a chest X-ray, pelvic X-ray and finally peritoneal lavage.

Management of multiple injuries is complicated and cannot be considered in detail in this chapter.

After ensuring adequate ventilation and an adequate blood pressure, a collar should be positioned in unconscious patients until the cervical spine has been X-rayed. If resuscitation does *not* result in a normal blood pressure (systolic > 100 mmHg) and pulse rate (< 125/min), then a more senior colleague should be consulted. Shock and immediate management of other injuries take priority over the management of the head injury, because if hypoxia and hypotension are present on arrival at the neurosurgical unit, the patient will almost certainly die. At this stage, after resuscitation is complete, the patient's level of consciousness should be assessed and recorded. The Glasgow Coma Scale (Teasdale and Jennett, 1974) has been widely adopted and is easy for nursing and medical staff to use. Repeated observations of the motor response, verbal performance and eye opening can be easily plotted on a chart (Figure 3.3). The history of the patient's level of responsiveness should be obtained from relatives, ambulance men or any other attendants to determine whether or not any deterioration has taken place since the injury, and this should also be recorded. In children the Glasgow Coma Scale has been modified (Simpson and Reilly, 1982) to take account of the normal reduced score in younger age groups.

At this stage other causes of coma should be considered. If it is obviously a head injury, then there is no problem. However, sometimes a patient falls during a seizure or while drunk, and the injury may be the result of another disease. Examples include epilepsy, elevated ICP from other intracranial lesions, diabetes, uraemia, hepatic failure, drugs or alcohol. The examination should record injuries to the scalp, eyes, ears, nose and face. The neurological examination can be brief and should include the pupillary reactions and the motor responses of each limb (to command if conscious and to pain if in coma). A decision should then be made about which X-rays (if any) should be performed urgently. All head-injured patients in coma should have a skull X-ray, as well as X-rays of the cervical spine and chest. As indicated at the outset, the majority of patients are not in coma and cervical spine and chest X-rays are only required if clinically indicated. Skull X-rays are useful because the presence of a skull fracture greatly increases the risk of an intracranial haematoma. Routine X-rays of the skull of all patients with head injury would be both unnecessary and expensive. Several studies have shown that some patients are

**Figure 3.3:** Glasgow Coma Chart. Note that the motor response is divided into five components. In assessing patients the flexor response should be subdivided into normal flexion and spastic flexion

INSTITUTE OF NEUROLOGICAL SCIENCES, GLASGOW

OBSERVATION CHART

SGH 172

| | | | DATE | | | | | | | | | | | | | | | | | | | | | | | | | | | | | | |
|---|---|---|---|---|---|---|---|---|---|---|---|---|---|---|---|---|---|---|---|---|---|---|---|---|---|---|---|---|---|---|---|---|---|
| NAME | | | | | | | | | | | | | | | | | | | | | | | | | | | | | | | | | |
| RECORD No. | | | TIME | | | | | | | | | | | | | | | | | | | | | | | | | | | | | | |
| **C** | Eyes open | Spontaneously | | | | | | | | | | | | | | | | | | | | | | | | | | | | | | Eyes closed by swelling = C |
| **O** | | To speech | | | | | | | | | | | | | | | | | | | | | | | | | | | | | | |
| | | To pain | | | | | | | | | | | | | | | | | | | | | | | | | | | | | | |
| **M** | | None | | | | | | | | | | | | | | | | | | | | | | | | | | | | | | |
| **A** | Best verbal response | Orientated | | | | | | | | | | | | | | | | | | | | | | | | | | | | | | Endotracheal tube or tracheostomy = T |
| | | Confused | | | | | | | | | | | | | | | | | | | | | | | | | | | | | | |
| **S** | | Inappropriate Words | | | | | | | | | | | | | | | | | | | | | | | | | | | | | | |
| | | Incomprehensible Sounds | | | | | | | | | | | | | | | | | | | | | | | | | | | | | | |
| **C** | | None | | | | | | | | | | | | | | | | | | | | | | | | | | | | | | |
| **A** | Best motor response | Obey commands | | | | | | | | | | | | | | | | | | | | | | | | | | | | | | Usually record the best arm response |
| | | Localise pain | | | | | | | | | | | | | | | | | | | | | | | | | | | | | | |
| **L** | | Flexion to pain | | | | | | | | | | | | | | | | | | | | | | | | | | | | | | |
| **E** | | Extension to pain | | | | | | | | | | | | | | | | | | | | | | | | | | | | | | |
| | | None | | | | | | | | | | | | | | | | | | | | | | | | | | | | | | |

more likely to have a fracture than others; guidelines for skull X-ray are set out in the Appendix. In addition, recent studies have suggested that headache and vomiting, and long and deep scalp lacerations are also commonly associated with skull fracture and should be added to the guidelines. They have therefore been included in the Appendix although not in the original published guidelines.

## Risk of haematoma

One in four adult patients in A&E who are not orientated and have a skull fracture will have a haematoma (Table 3.3). *All these patients should be referred for a CT scan.* If there is no skull fracture and the patient is fully orientated on admission to hospital, the risk of a haematoma is only 1 in 6000. These patients can be sent home with a caring relative or friend and with instructions to return if new symptoms develop. Patients with intermediate levels of risk (Table 3.3) should be admitted to hospital for observation.

**Table 3.3:** Risks of traumatic intracranial haematomas in adult patients in A&E (Mendelow *et al.*, 1983)

| Risk factors | Risk of haematoma |
|---|---|
| No skull fracture: | |
| orientated | 1:5983 |
| not orientated | 1:121 |
| Skull fracture | |
| orientated | 1:32 |
| not orientated | 1:4 |

There is controversy about whether or not to admit for observation patients with a brief history of unconsciousness or amnesia. Although this is still recommended in some texts (Potter, 1984), the likelihood of a haematoma is very small if the patient has recovered completely to a fully oriented state and has no fracture. These patients do not require admission to hospital. This policy would save many unnecessary admissions if it was widely accepted, and the guidelines clearly indicate that if a patient is fully conscious and oriented, then admission is *not* required. It has to be acknowledged that a few patients will return with a haematoma, but the risk is so small for adults that agreement was reached when the guidelines were drawn up. It should be stressed that if such patients have had any indication for skull X-ray, then this should be checked first, because a skull fracture, even if the patient is oriented, carries a 1 in 32 risk of haematoma for adults in A&E. Different views on the value of skull X-ray have been expressed from North America where CT scanners are abundant and where the initial radiology in a head-injured patient is often a CT scan rather than a skull X-ray. Obviously, if there is free access to CT scanning for casualty patients, then the skull X-ray step can be omitted. However, in most countries CT scanning is *not* readily available for all head-injured patients, and the skull X-ray must remain a useful diagnostic step. It should be stressed that these guidelines only apply to adult patients (15 years and over) because the data on level of consciousness in children are difficult to interpret. Although the same principles may indeed apply to children, as yet no clear guidelines have emerged. It is probably safer to err on the side of caution and to admit children for observation if there is any doubt and certainly if there is any clouding of consciousness.

## MANAGEMENT AFTER THE INITIAL ASSESSMENT AND X-RAYS

After the initial assessment and resuscitation, the patient can either be:

(1) referred to a neurological centre;
(2) admitted to a general ward for observation;
(3) sent home with a caring relative.

It is suggested that the guidelines set out in the Appendix should be displayed prominently in the A&E or Casualty Department. They define which of these three options should be chosen for an individual patient.

Patients who have a low risk of developing a haematoma (Table 3.3) can be sent home with a caring friend or relative. That person should be told that the patient must be brought back to the hospital if there is any deterioration in the level of consciousness, any vomiting or any other abnormality. Patients with intermediate levels of risk (no skull fracture, but not orientated, i.e. confused or worse; or with a skull fracture but still fully orientated) should be admitted for observation to a general ward where nursing staff have been instructed in the use of the Glasgow Coma Scale. Any deterioration is recorded and the patient should immediately be transferred to a Regional Neurosurgical Unit provided there is no other cause such as hypoxia or hypertension.

If it is clear from the initial assessment that the patient has a high risk (1 in 4) of developing an intracranial haematoma, then transfer to the Regional Neurosurgical Unit is advised after consultation with a neurosurgeon. In most cases this will result in the patient having a CT scan. If CT scanning is readily available in the referring hospital, then all these high-risk patients should be scanned provided that this does not induce prolonged delays. Usually this can be done within 2 hours in the United Kingdom, so that it is very seldom necessary to perform emergency burr holes or surgery in the original hospital. On very rare occasions, when a patient has been alert and talking and subsequently the level of consciousness has deteriorated with the development of a fixed dilated pupil and a boggy scalp mass on the same side, and where transfer to a neurosurgical unit would result in delay of more than 2 hours, then a temporal burr hole should be performed on the side of the abnormal pupil. If an extradural haemorrhage is encountered, then it should be evacuated by enlarging the burr hole to form a craniectomy using bone rongeurs. This life-saving procedure is very rarely necessary but should be considered in the particular circumstances which are outlined above. Exploratory burr holes should *not* be performed routinely in patients who have been in coma from the moment of the impact because the outcome is no better for such patients and because some haematomas will be missed: an urgent CT scan will prove more useful. The other categories of patient to be transferred for neurosurgical care are those at risk of developing infection (meningitis or brain abscess). These are patients with compound depressed fractures, penetrating wounds or cerebrospinal fluid leaks (categories 5 and 6 of the Guidelines for Consultation with a Neurosurgeon).

## Dangers of transfer

Before any patient is transferred it is essential that they have been adequately resuscitated so that on arrival in the neurosurgical unit their blood pressure and respiration are normal. Failure to ensure this has repeatedly been shown to result in poor outcome. Nevertheless, hypoxic and shocked patients with multiple injuries continue to be referred by junior staff because of concern about coma. This dangerous practice should not be allowed to continue.

## Observation in a general ward

The majority of head-injured admissions will be observed for 24 to 48 hours in general wards, and then discharged home. If the guidelines are followed, then these will be patients without a skull fracture who are confused and their confusion should clear within 6 to 8 hours. If the confusion persists beyond this period, then they too should be referred for a CT scan (Guidelines category 4). Other patients will be those with a skull fracture who are fully oriented. If such patients remain oriented, they can be sent home the next day. If they develop confusion, they then should be referred for a CT scan. A short period of concussion is *not* an indication for admission to hospital provided that the patient has recovered fully and is oriented when seen. Longer periods of concussion (> 5 minutes) may be associated with diffuse axonal injury (DAI), and may require admission to reduce the frequency of the post-concussion syndrome.

There is a particular problem with *children* in that it is not possible to establish full orientation as can be done in an adult. They should therefore be observed in the hospital even if the period of initial concussion *is* less than 5 minutes. Monitoring the level of consciousness in children should be with the Paediatric Coma Scale (Simpson and Reilly, 1982).

## MANAGEMENT IN A NEUROSURGICAL UNIT

The main reason for early transfer of patients after initial resuscitation is to detect intracranial haematomas. Most of these patients will require CT scanning (although in centres where CT scanning is not available, angiography may be indicated). Many of these patients are restless, and sedation may be required to facilitate investigation. It is dangerous to sedate a recently head-injured patient, because sedative drugs reduce respiratory drive which results in hypercapnia and elevated intracranial pressure. If a patient does require anaesthesia, then a full general anaesthetic given by a neuroanaesthetist is the safest technique. This is because intubation and ventilation or hyperventilation are often required. This prevents an acute rise in intracranial pressure, and if the patient subsequently requires a craniotomy or intracranial pressure monitoring, they can then be moved straight into the operating theatre.

Fortunately, sedation is seldom required with modern CT scanners because of the faster speed of scanning. Only limited views without contrast injection are needed in most head-injured patients, so that the whole procedure can be completed within 5 minutes.

## Investigations

(1) *Plain X-rays*. Skull X-rays are usually taken in the referring hospitals, but should always be sent on to the neurosurgical unit. These may show the expected fracture (Figure 3.4) or the shift of a calcified pineal. Air in the anterior fossa or in the ventricular system may indicate a basal skull fracture.

(2) *CT scanning*. Many more lesions are seen on CT scan than were known to occur in the pre-CT era. Not all these lesions (especially intracerebral haematomas) require evacuation. If a patient has clearly deteriorated, then there is no doubt that a haematoma should be evacuated (Figure 3.5a), but if a patient is still able to talk or is even improving but has a haematoma, especially if it is intracerebral (Figure 3.5c), then a conservative/expectant policy should be adopted. In this situation, ICP monitoring is useful:

— if the ICP is greater than 30 mmHg, then the clot should be removed;

— if less than 20 mmHg, it should be left; and

— if 20–30 mmHg, then a further period of monitoring should clarify the situation.

(3) *MRI scanning*. Recent studies of head-injured patients have indicated that twice as many lesions can be detected on MRI as on CT scanning (Figure 3.6). In particular DAI, which does not show up well on CT scan, can be seen on MR imaging. Another advantage of MR imaging is its ability to demonstrate haematomas in the same way as a CT scan (Figures 3.5a, b and c).

(4) *Angiography*. If the imaging techniques referred to above are not available as emergency procedures, then angiography may be required. Limited films are needed in head-injured patients, and in fact a single unilateral carotid injection on a Townes view of the skull will demonstrate shift and a surface haematoma if present.

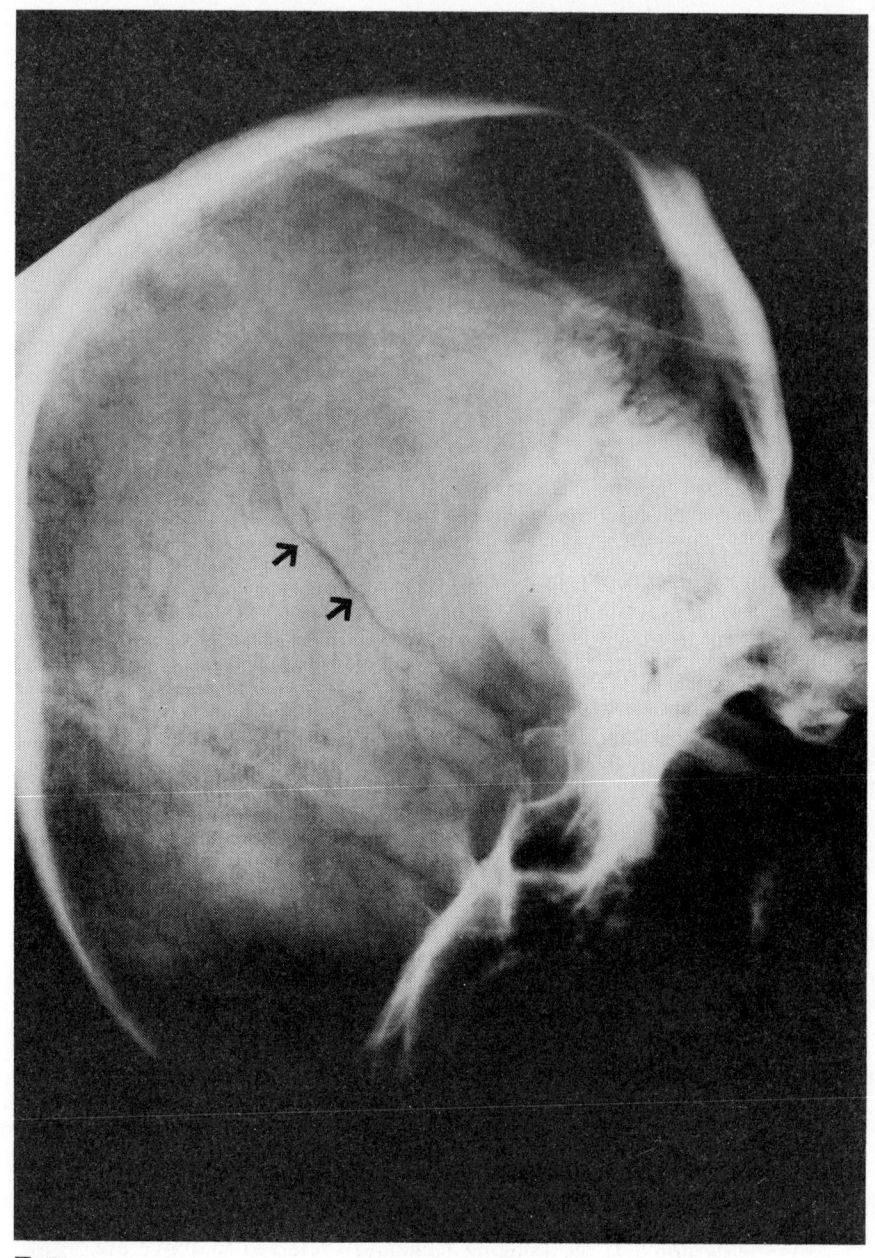

**Figure 3.4:** Skull X-ray showing a linear fracture (arrow)

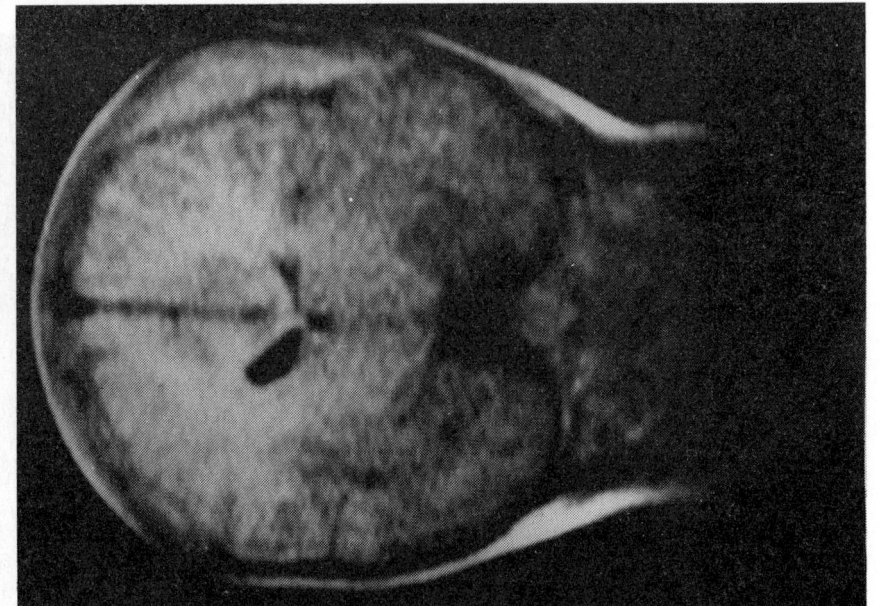

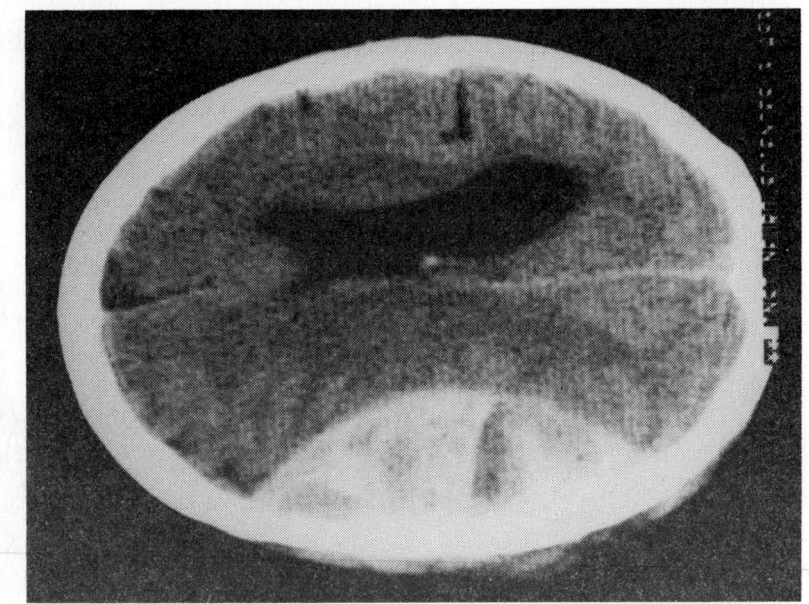

**Figure 3.5:** CT scans (left) and MR images (right) of (a) extradural haematoma

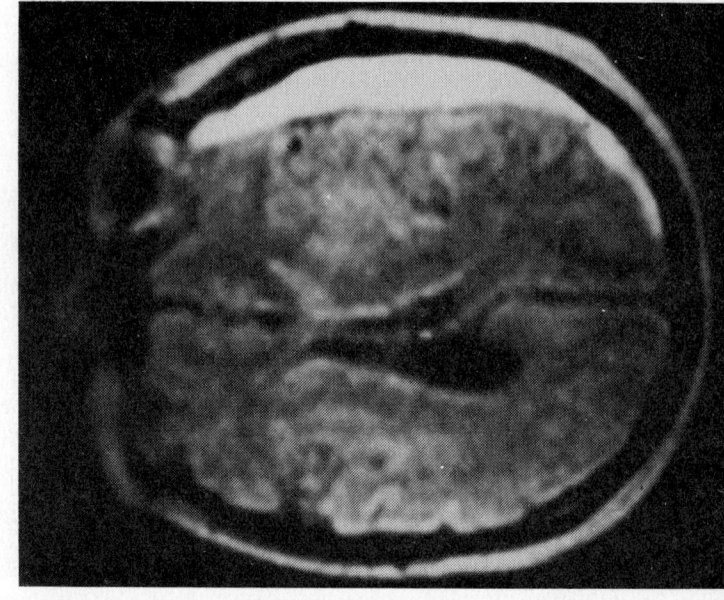

**Figure 3.5:** (b) acute subdural haematoma

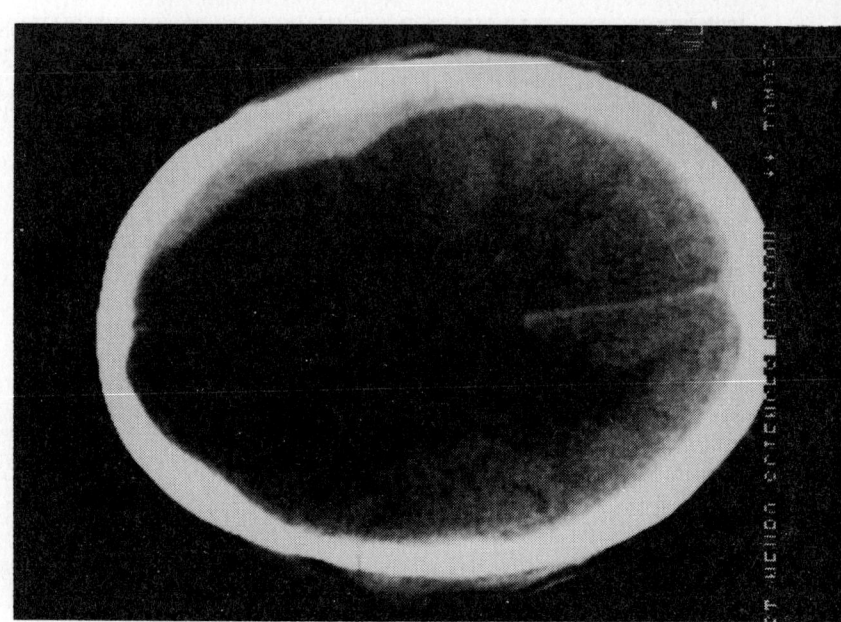

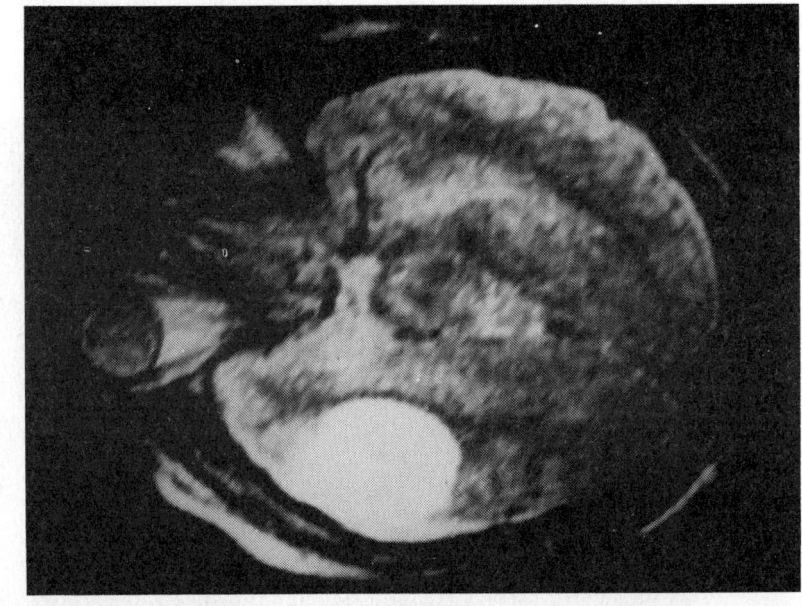

**Figure 3.5:** (c) intracerebral haematoma

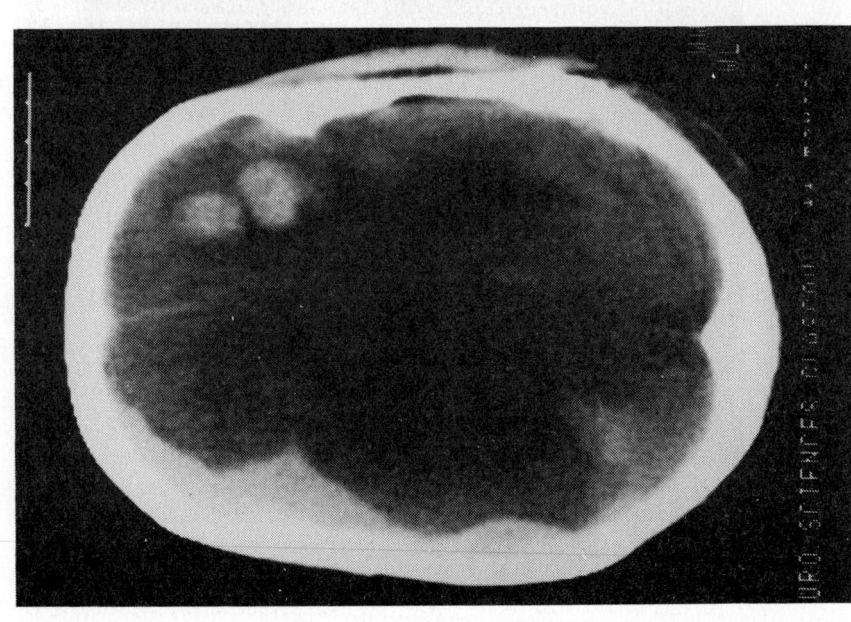

**Figure 3.6:** MR image in a patient with diffuse axonal injury. The lesions appear as high-density (white) areas which were not visible on CT scan. (From Jenkins *et al*. (1986), with permission.)

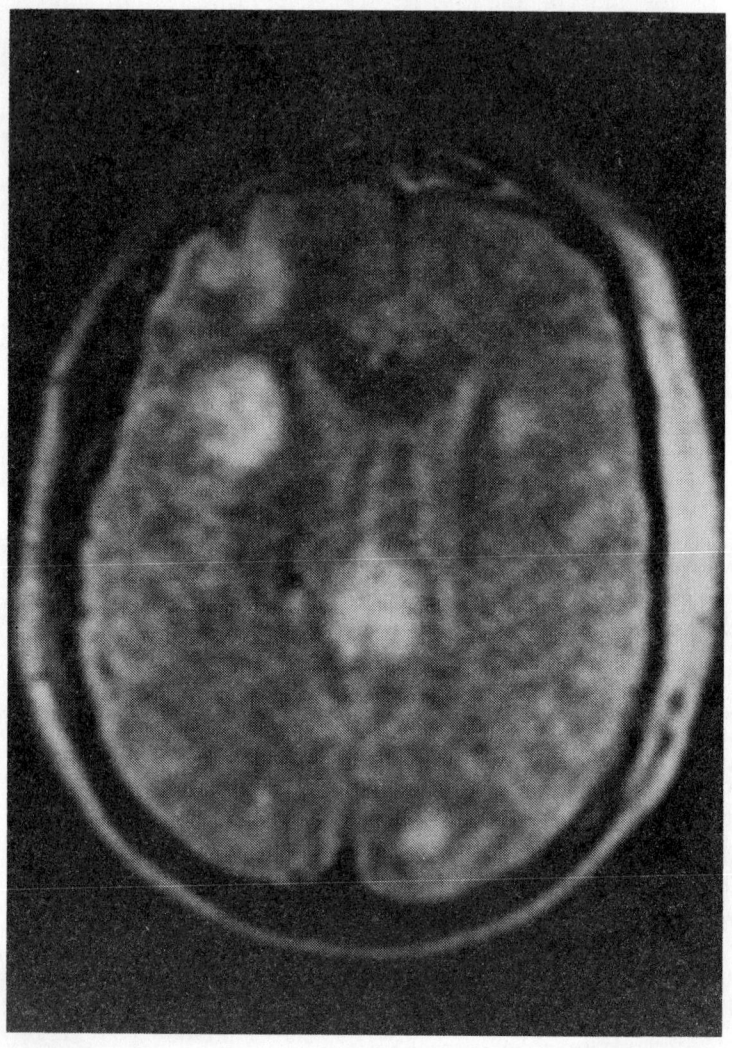

## Observation for haematomas

Most patients admitted to neurosurgical units according to these guidelines will have had a CT scan, and if a haematoma is present they will fall into one of three categories:

(1) require urgent operative removal;
(2) no definite indication for operation: intracranial pressure monitoring indicated;
(3) the patient's clinical condition is so good that no treatment is required.

Patients in this last category will usually be observed for 24 to 48 hours, and if stable can be transferred back to the district hospital. Patients in categories 1 and 2 are dealt with later under operative treatment.

## Prevention of infection

Two categories of patient are at risk: those with CSF leaks, and those with compound depressed fractures.

Patients with *CSF leaks* should be treated with a penicillin and sulphonamide for 5 days. If the leak stops (as do the vast majority), no further treatment is required.

Patients with *compound depressed fractures* should also receive prophylactic antibiotic treatment with penicillin and a sulphonamide. Classic teaching is that the wound should be debrided, and the dura repaired if it is disrupted. There is a trend to treat some of the non-missile injuries with compound depressed fractures conservatively: if the wound is clean, and fragments are not indriven deeply, then good primary skin closure with antibiotic cover is not associated with a higher infection rate. If meningitis or a brain abscess develops, then high-dosage intravenous antibiotic treatment is required with penicillin (12 Mu per day) and chloramphenicol (500 mg 6-hourly).

## Management of severe head injuries in coma

Irrespective of the presence or absence of haematomas some patients will remain in coma, and half of all patients who remain in coma for more than 6 hours will die no matter what type of treatment is given. Although elevated ICP is associated with a higher morbidity and mortality treatment aimed at reducing ICP has not been shown to improve outcome. In a randomised control trial of patients with severe head injury, Ward *et al.* (1986) showed that barbiturates do not improve the outcome. In an analysis of 1000 severely head-injured patients, Jennett *et al.* (1980) showed that even when the severity of the injury was taken into account, the use of steroids and tracheostomy did not affect outcome, and patients undergoing mechanical ventilation actually fared worse than expected. Subsequently, Braakman *et al.* (1983) showed in a prospective randomised controlled trial that dexamethasone did not improve the outcome of these patients compared with placebo. Although there is enthusiasm for other types of pharmacological treatment for severe head injury, there is as yet no proof that any of these agents should be used in clinical practice. Examples include GAMA hydroxybutyric acid, dimethyl sulphoxide, isoflurane and more recently calcium antagonists. Despite the despondency which the results of these trials engender in all those called upon to treat these patients, there is agreement that good intensive care, with attention to the airway and prevention of extracranial insults, is an essential and effective component of head-injury management. The difficult dividing line to draw is that between good cardiorespiratory care and over-treatment. The goal must remain: maintenance of normoxia and a good cerebral perfusion pressure at all times.

## Operative treatment

(1) *ICP Monitoring.* ICP is usually monitored by a right frontal burr hole. A ventricular catheter can be connected to a pressure transducer for continuous recording (Figure 3.7). Recent studies have shown that subdural screw devices are unreliable. Similarly, open-ended subdural catheters are inaccurate although subdural catheters with inbuilt transducers are as reliable as ventricular catheters. These catheter-tipped transducers in the subdural spaces have the advantage that ventricular puncture is avoided, thereby reducing the risk of epilepsy, infection and haematoma. Monitoring is usually continued for 2 to 5 days. Longer periods of monitoring expose the patients to unnecessarily increased risks of infection.

Elevated ICP (> 30 mmHg) with an intracranial haematoma is an indication for urgent craniotomy provided that there is no other cause for the raised ICP such as hypoxia.

(2) *Evacuation of haematomas.* These are best removed via a large craniotomy positioned over the site of the haematoma. Rapid decompression should be provided as early as possible during the operation, even via the first burr hole, which should therefore be suitably positioned. Surface haematomas are well delineated and can be completely removed. Intracerebral haematomas and contusions are more difficult and considerable judgement is required in deciding how much surrounding brain to decompress. There is no good evidence that a lobectomy (as a form of internal decompression) is superior to more conservative surgery (removal of just the obvious haematoma). It is for this reason that ICP monitoring is recommended for patients with 'occult' intracerebral haematomas: many of these lesions on CT scan resolve spontaneously without any period of raised ICP. Acute subdural haematomas cannot be removed adequately through burr holes, and should rather be evacuated through a large craniotomy.

(3) *Compound depressed fractures.*

   (a) *Missile injuries.* There is universal agreement that these lesions should be debrided, all bone fragments should be removed from the surface and the dura should be repaired.

   (b) *Non-missile injuries.* Where a decision has been taken to operate, the wound is cleaned and the skin edges are trimmed appropriately. Bone fragments are removed and cleaned and can be replaced to avoid a subsequent cranioplasty. The dura is repaired after removing any indriven dirt, hair or foreign body.

   (c) *CSF leaks.* When a CSF leak persists for more than one week, where there is an aerocoele or if there has been an episode of meningitis, then a bifrontal craniotomy is performed for an anterior fossa repair, and, less frequently, a subtemporal craniectomy for a middle fossa repair. The fracture and dural tear are identified intradurally and artificial dura is layered over the site and fixed in position with tissue glue.

**Figure 3.7:** Intracranial pressure monitoring via a frontal ventricular catheter. (Modified from Jennett and Teasdale (1981), with permission.)

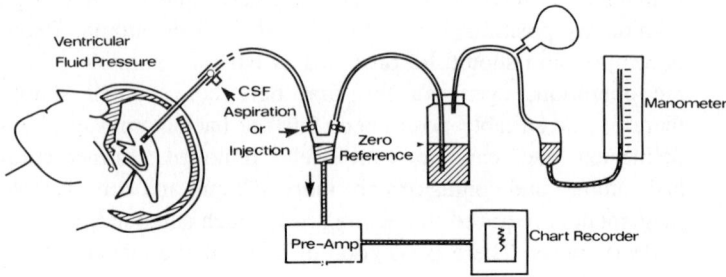

## LATE COMPLICATIONS OF HEAD INJURY

### 1. Epilepsy

The risk of developing late post-traumatic epilepsy after a non-missile head injury can be determined from tables published by Jennett (1975). For compound depressed fractures these risks are summarised in Figure 3.8.

### 2. Chronic subdural haematomas

After one to two weeks subdural clots become liquid and patients may present with confusion or focal neurological signs. Sometimes there is no history of previous head injury. Small lesions in patients with headache and no focal neurological signs will sometimes respond well to medical treatment with dexamethasone. Larger lesions can be washed out via one or two burr holes. Recent evidence suggests that post-operative closed system drainage of the subdural space for 48 hours improves the results.

### 3. Permanent brain damage

A distressingly high number of patients who survive their head

**Figure 3.8:** The frequency with which different combinations of factors occurred is displayed below the incidence of late epilepsy associated with each combination (three factors of four available). (From Jennett (1975), with permission.)

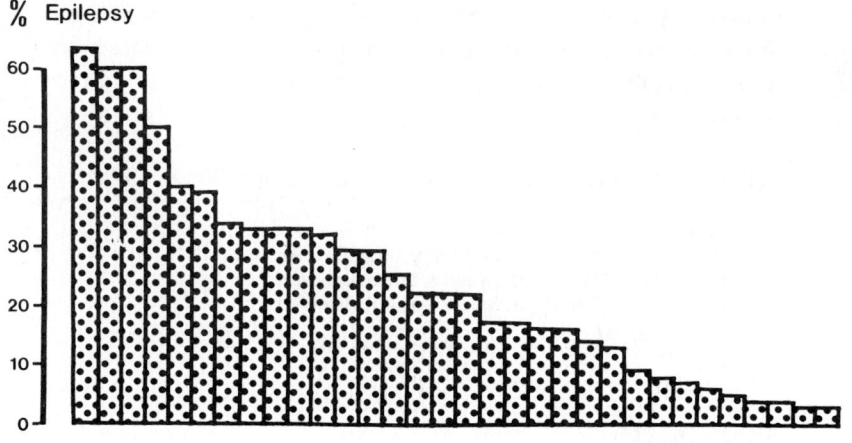

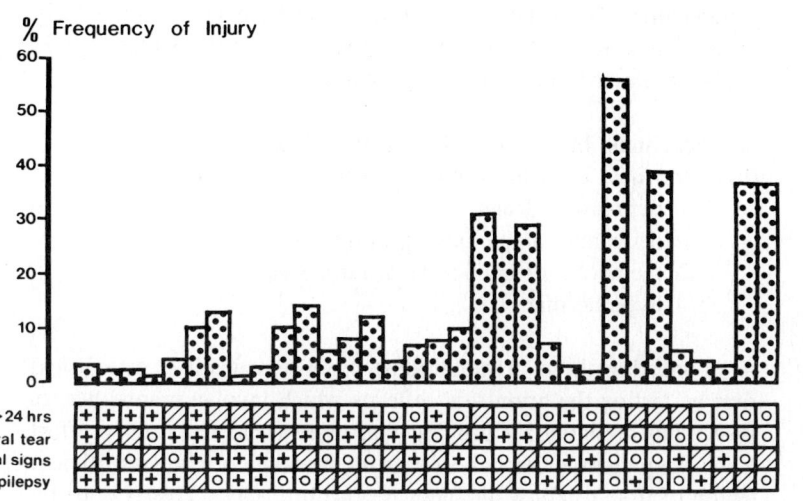

injury remain severely disabled. The goal of head-injury management is to reduce this number as well as to reduce mortality. The outcome is usefully measured on a 5-point scale described by Jennett and Bond (1975) and referred to as the Glasgow Outcome Scale (Table 3.4). It is now possible to predict the eventual outcome on this scale at early stages in the course of a head injury. This has been made possible by referring to the Data Bank of Severe Head Injuries, held in Glasgow.

**Table 3.4:** Glasgow Outcome Scale (Jennett and Bond, 1975)

| | |
|---|---|
| Death | |
| Vegetative state: | persistently unconscious |
| Severe disability: | conscious but dependent |
| Moderate disability: | independent but disabled |
| Good recovery | |

## BRAIN DEATH

Unfortunately, those who care for severe head injury will be faced with patients who, despite all treatment, become brain dead while on a ventilator. The criteria for brain death have now been widely accepted (Jennett, 1983). Certain preconditions must exist *before* applying the criteria. These preconditions are:

(a) there must be irreversible structural brain damage;
(b) there must be apnoeic coma which is *not* due to
    (i) depressant drugs,
    (ii) neuromuscular blocking agents,
    (iii) metabolic or endocrine disturbances,
    (iv) hypothermia.

After meeting these preconditions, brainstem death is established first by testing the brainstem reflexes which involve cranial nerves II–X, and secondly by proving that there is no respiratory effort when the patient is disconnected from the respirator for a sufficient length of time to allow an adequate rise in $P_a CO_2$. This is done by disconnecting the patient and inserting a fine catheter down the endotracheal tube and delivering oxygen through it at 6 litres/min; the patient may have to remain disconnected for as long as 10 minutes because the rise in $P_a CO_2$ is slow (about 2 mmHg/min). Arterial blood gases should be checked at the end of the period of apnoea to ensure that the $P_aCO_2$ has *exceeded* 50 mmHg. If blood gas analysis is not available, the alternative procedure is to supply the ventilator with pure oxygen for 10 minutes (pre-oxygenation), then with 5% $CO_2$ in oxygen for 5 minutes, and *then* to *disconnect* the ventilator for 10 minutes while delivering oxygen at 6 litres/min via a catheter in the trachea. These findings should be confirmed independently and recorded on a proforma (Table 3.5) by two doctors, at least one of whom should be a consultant (Code of Practice, 1979).

**Table 3.5**: Brain-death criteria

| *Preconditions*<br>Nature of irremediable brain damage | Time of event<br>leading to coma | |
| --- | --- | --- |
| Dr A _____ | | |
| Dr B _____ | | |
| Do you consider that apnoeic coma is due to: | Dr A | Dr B |
|     Depressant drugs | _____ | |
|     Neuromuscular blocking<br>      (relaxant) drugs | _____ | |
|     Hypothermia | _____ | |
|     Metabolic or endocrine disturbances | _____ | |
| *Tests for absence of brain-stem function* | | |
| Is there evidence of: | Dr A | Dr B |
|     Pupil reaction to light | _____ | |
|     Corneal reflex | _____ | |
|     Eye movements with cold caloric test | _____ | |
|     Cranial nerve motor responses | _____ | |
|     Gag reflex | _____ | |
|     Respiratory movements on<br>      disconnection from ventilator to<br>      allow adequate rise in $P_aCO_2$ | _____ | |
| Date and time of first testing _____ | | |
| Date and time of second testing _____ | | |

*Dr A*                     *Dr B*

Signature _____     Signature _____

Status _____     Status _____

## APPENDIX

Guidelines (Neurosurgical Department, Institute of Neurological Sciences, Glasgow)

---

**Criteria for consultation about patients with recent head injury**

1. Fractured skull
      with confusion or worse impairment of consciousness, or
      with focal neurological signs, or
      with fits, or
      with any other neurological symptoms or signs
2. Coma continuing after resuscitation — even if no skull fracture
3. Deterioration in level of consciousness or other neurological signs
4. Confusion or other neurological disturbances persisting for more than 6–8 hours, even if there is no skull fracture
5. Compound depressed fracture of the vault of the skull
6. Suspected fracture of base of skull (CSF rhinorrhoea or otorrhoea, bilateral orbital haematoma, mastoid haematoma) or other penetrating injury (gunshot, etc.)

   Patients in categories 1–3 should be referred urgently

   - Note: In all cases the diagnosis and initial treatment of serious extracranial injuries takes priority over transfer to the neurosurgical unit.

*Management of head-injured patients in coma or with possible multiple injuries*

1. Assess for respiratory insufficiency, for shock, and for internal injuries, especially after a high-velocity injury, e.g. a road traffic accident.
2. Perform: (a) chest X-ray; (b) blood gas estimation; (c) cervical spine X-ray; (d) other investigations as relevant.
3. Appropriate treatment may include:
      Intubate (e.g. if airways obstructed or threatened)
      Ventilate (e.g. cyanosis, $P_aO_2 < 60$ mmHg, $P_aCO_2 > 45$ mmHg)
      Commence IV infusion (1500 ml/24 h *and* colloid or blood if shocked to maintain BP)
      Mannitol, only after consultation with neurosurgeon
      Application of cervical collar or cervical traction
      Immobilisation of fractures, treatment of internal injuries
4. If accepted for transfer the patient should be accompanied by personnel able to insert or to re-position endotracheal tube, and to initiate or to maintain ventilation.

**Guidelines for the management of patients with recent head injury**

*Criteria for skull X-ray after recent head injury*

Clinical judgement is necessary but the following criteria are helpful:

1. Loss of consciousness or amnesia at any time
2. Neurological symptoms or signs (including headache and vomiting)
3. Cerebrospinal fluid or blood from the nose or ear

4. Suspected penetrating injury
5. Scalp bruising, swelling and/or long deep lacerations
6. Difficulty in assessing the patient (i.e. alcohol intoxication, epilepsy, children)

*Criteria for admission of adults to hospital*

1. Confusion or any other depression of the level of consciousness at the time of examination
2. Skull fracture
3. Neurological symptoms or signs
4. Difficulty in assessing the patient, e.g. alcohol, epilepsy
5. Other medical conditions — e.g. haemophilia
6. The patient's social conditions or lack of a responsible adult/relative

Post-traumatic amnesia or unconsciousness with full recovery is not necessarily an indication for admission.

Patients sent home should receive advice to return immediately if there is any deterioration.

Adapted from Harrogate Seminar Report 8, *The management of acute head injury*, DHSS, London, 1983, and 'Guidelines for the initial management after head injury in adults', *Brit. Med. J.* 1984, *288*, 983–5.

## ACKNOWLEDGEMENTS

I would like to thank Professor J.H. Adams and Professor D.L. Graham for providing Figure 3.2, Dr. D. Hadley for providing MR images, and the Department of Medical Illustration of the Institute of Neurological Sciences in Glasgow for preparing the artwork. Thanks also to Anne Semple (Department of Neurosurgery, University of Glasgow) for preparing the typescript.

## FURTHER READING

'A Group of Neurosurgeons' (1984) Guidelines for initial management after head injury in adults. *Brit. Med. J.* 288, 983–5
Braakman, R., Schouten, H.J.A. and Blaan-Van Dishock, M. (1983) Megadose steroids in severe head injury: results of a prospective double blind clinical trial. *J. Neurosurg.* 58, 326–30
Brookes, M.T., Mendelow, A.D., MacMillan, R. *et al.* (1986) Which head injured patients have a skull fracture? *Arch, Emer. Med. 31*, 41–92
Galbraith, S. and Teasdale, G.M. (1982) Head injuries. In: R.C.G. Russell (ed.) *Recent advances in surgery*, Churchill Livingstone, Edinburgh, 71–84.
Gentleman, D. and Jennett, B. (1981) Hazards of inter-hospital transfer of comatose head injured patients. *Lancet ii*, 853–5

Jennett, B. (1975) *Epilepsy after non-missile head injury*, 2nd edn. Heinemann, London

Jennett, B. (1983) Brain death 1983. *Practitioner* 227, 451–4

Jennett, B. and Bond, M. (1975) Assessment of outcome after severe brain damage. *Lancet i*, 480

Jennett, B., Teasdale, G.M. and Fry, J. (1980) Treatment for severe head injury. *J. Neurol. Neurosurg. Psychiat.* 43, 289–95

Jennett, B. and Teasdale, G.M. (1981) *Management of head injuries*. F.A. Davis, Philadelphia

Kohi, Y.M., Mendelow, A.D., Teasdale, G.M. *et al.* (1984) Extracranial insults and outcome in patients with acute head injury — relationship to the Glasgow Coma Scale. *Injury 16*, 25–9

Mendelow, A.D., Campbell, D.A., Jeffrey, R.R. *et al.* (1982) Admission after mild head injury: benefits and costs. *Brit. Med. J.* 285, 1530–2

Mendelow, A.D., Teasdale, G.M. and Jennett, B. (1983) Risks of intracranial haematoma in head injured adults. *Brit. Med. J.* 287, 1173–6

Miller, J.D. and Becker, D.P. (1982) Secondary insults to the injured brain. *J. Roy. Coll. Surg. Edinburgh 27*, 292–8

Potter, J.M. (1984) *The practical management of head injuries*, 4th edn. Lloyd Luke, London, p. 25

Seelig, J.M., Becker, D.P., Miller, J.D. *et al.* (1981) Traumatic acute subdural haematomas; major mortality reduction in comatose patients treated within four hours. *N. Engl. J. Med. 304*, 1511–18

Simpson, D. and Reilly, P. (1982) Paediatric Coma Scale. *Lancet ii*, 450

Teasdale, G.M. (1984) Head injuries are badly managed in accident and emergency departments and neurosurgeons are partly to blame. *Arch. Emerg. Med. 3*, 123–34

Teasdale, G.M. and Jennett, B. (1974) Assessment of coma and impaired consciousness: a practical scale. *Lancet ii*, 81–4

Ward, J.D., Miller, J.D., Choi, S.C. *et al.* (1986) Failure of prophylactic barbiturate coma in the prevention of death due to uncontrollable intracranial hypertension in patients with severe head injury. In J.D. Miller, G.M. Teasdale, J.O. Rowan, S.L. Galbraith and A.D. Mendelow (eds.) *ICP VI* Springer-Verlag, Berlin and Heidelberg

Working Party on Behalf of the Health Departments of Great Britain and Northern Ireland (1979) *The removal of cadaveric organs for transplantation. A Code of Practice*, Her Majesty's Stationery Office, London

# 4

# Subarachnoid Haemorrhage

A. David Mendelow

## INTRODUCTION

Patients with spontaneous subarachnoid haemorrhage (SAH) may present in several different ways. These range from the 'warning leak' to coma or even death. Aneurysms are the commonest cause of SAH, which may also result from a ruptured arteriovenous malformation (AVM), from a tumour or from a blood dyscrasia. In addition to causing SAH, aneurysms may cause spontaneous intracerebral haemorrhage. More frequent use of the computer tomographic (CT) scanner now brings a greater number of such cases to light.

The outlook for patients with a ruptured intracranial aneurysm is grim. Left untreated, more than half will be dead within a year, yet operation now offers the prospect of a cure for at least 90% of patients who survive the initial ictus. Because of this very high early morbidity and mortality a patient with a suspected SAH should be assumed to have an aneurysm until proved otherwise. The burden of primary health care is therefore to diagnose and to refer for urgent treatment any patient who is suspected of having had a subarachnoid haemorrhage. The management objective is to identify and to treat those patients who have survived their first haemorrhage, and who are at risk of rebleeding.

The first problem therefore is to diagnose the SAH. Because the clinical presentation varies from the warning leak to death, the clinician must maintain a low threshold for its diagnosis. Because other conditions may mimic SAH (e.g. epilepsy, occlusive stroke or meningitis), the diagnosis should be made by performing a lumbar puncture or CT scan as soon as possible. The choice of investigation is discussed in more detail later. The second problem is to find the cause of the haemorrhage. Four-vessel angiography will correctly diagnose an aneurysm or an AVM. It is important to examine the whole cerebral circulation because a quarter of patients with SAH will have multiple aneurysms, and because some patients with an AVM may have an associated aneurysm. Surgical treatment cannot be planned without this knowledge. The third problem is to prevent rebleeding. With aneurysms, the surest way is to clip the neck of the ruptured aneurysm.

Unfortunately, operative treatment may produce the fourth problem, which is cerebral ischaemia due to vasospasm. Crompton (1964) found that ischaemic brain damage occurred in 70% of patients who died following SAH. This initially led many surgeons to recommend delaying operative intervention because clinical ischaemia occurred less frequently in patients operated upon after the second week. However, many patients who were otherwise in good condition died from rebleeding during the waiting period. There has been a swing back to earlier surgery to avoid the risk of rebleeding because treatment is now available for ischaemia due to arterial spasm once the aneurysm has been clipped. It is clear that early surgery in well patients is as safe in the first few days as it is after delaying for seven or more days. There can therefore be no justification for exposing patients, who have recovered well, to the risk of bleeding during an unnecessarily prolonged pre-operative waiting period. The contribution that the neuroanaesthetist and the neuroradiologist have made to these improved surgical results cannot be overemphasised. Surgical techniques have also improved, and the prognosis of a patient with a ruptured aneurysm is now much better than previously (Sengupta and McAllister, 1986).

## EPIDEMIOLOGY

The incidence of SAH is between 4 and 20 per 100 000 per year. This range is in accord with the *rate of haemorrhage* from unruptured aneurysms, which is 1% per year. Given a *prevalence* of aneurysm of 1% in the general population (as is suggested from autopsy series), the expected *incidence* of new SAH due to aneurysm should be 10 per 100 000 per annum (i.e. 1% of 1% per annum). The predicted *rate of haemorrhage* from unruptured aneurysms and their *prevalence* therefore match up well with the *incidence* of new SAH in the general population. Once an aneurysm has ruptured, the risk of rebleeding is much higher. In a large series of patients treated with bed rest alone, approximately 30% of patients who survived their first haemorrhage rebled within 4 weeks. The risk of rebleeding continues at the rate of 3% per annum thereafter so that the cumulative risk is higher in younger patients. This 'age factor' applies to both ruptured and unruptured aneurysms, and must be considered when balancing the natural history against the risk of surgery.

The risk of haemorrhage from an unruptured arteriovenous malformation is between 2 and 3% per year, while from ruptured lesions the risk is 6% in the first year and 2% per year thereafter. In general, smaller lesions seem less likely to bleed.


## PATHOPHYSIOLOGY

At the time of the initial ictus, clinical studies have shown that there is a release of blood under arterial pressure into the subarachnoid space so that intracranial pressure (ICP) rises until it reaches the mean arterial blood pressure (MABP). This reduction in cerebral perfusion pressure (CPP) is probably what produces the ischaemic brain damage reported by Crompton (1964). *Experimental* studies have confirmed that this mechanism leads to a fall in cerebral blood flow (CBF) with histological evidence of ischaemic brain damage. Following the initial insult, there is a loss of autoregulation of CBF so that it becomes passively dependent upon the perfusion pressure. This has also been demonstrated *in patients* with SAH from ruptured aneurysms pre-, intra- and post-operatively, and has led clinicians to recognise that the maintenance of CPP is essential in these patients. This can be achieved by maintaining MABP or lowering ICP. During the initial period when autoregulation is lost, successful and permanent reversal of the neurological deficit associated with delayed cerebral ischaemia was achieved in 43 patients out of 58 using a combination of hypervolaemia and pharmacologically induced hypertension with dopamine (Kassell *et al.*, 1982). Any fall in MABP may lead to a fall in CBF with the development of focal neurological features. It should be added that a fall in CPP may also be the result of hydrocephalus with raised ICP, which can develop as a result of blood that blocks the subarachnoid spaces and the arachnoid villi. In these circumstances, drainage of the hydrocephalus (by catheter or ventriculo-peritoneal shunt) may increase CPP and this may then improve the clinical picture.

## CLINICAL PRESENTATION

The well-known clinical features of sudden severe occipital headache and meningism are familiar to all clinicians. Nevertheless, the presentation of SAH may vary from a single severe headache (the warning leak), through the classical clinical picture, to coma. Focal neurological signs such as hemiplegia or aphasia may result from reduced flow to the hemisphere. Localised compression of the third nerve by a posterior communicating artery aneurysm may produce a unilateral fixed dilated pupil with retro-ocular pain. It should also be remembered that epilepsy may be a manifestation of SAH in a quarter of patients, so that, if a patient complains of severe headache associated with the abrupt onset of epilepsy, then such a patient should be referred for urgent CT scanning.

### 1. Is it really a subarachnoid haemorrhage?

The mainstay of diagnosis of SAH has always been the lumbar puncture (LP). However, in some patients this may prove hazardous because it may lead to tentorial herniation or a medullary cone if there is a mass with raised ICP, or because it may reduce the tamponade effect of the brain on the fundus of the aneurysm and thereby LP may precipitate a rebleed. It is therefore recommended that patients with suspected SAH who are not oriented, who have papilloedema or who have focal neurological signs should first have a CT scan and not an LP. If this confirms the presence of blood (Figure 4.1), then the LP is obviously unnecessary. It is practically impossible to subject all cases of suspected SAH (especially with minor symptoms of the type described as a warning leak) to CT scanning, so LP must remain the primary investigation in the majority of patients (Figure 4.2). Furthermore, the delay in transporting these patients for a CT scan can lead to delay in the treatment of otherwise treatable conditions such as meningitis, which may mimic SAH. *There can be no reason to delay LP in patients with suspected SAH who are oriented and without focal signs and with no papilloedema.*

### 2. What is the cause of SAH?

If the diagnosis is made first on LP, then the patient should undergo

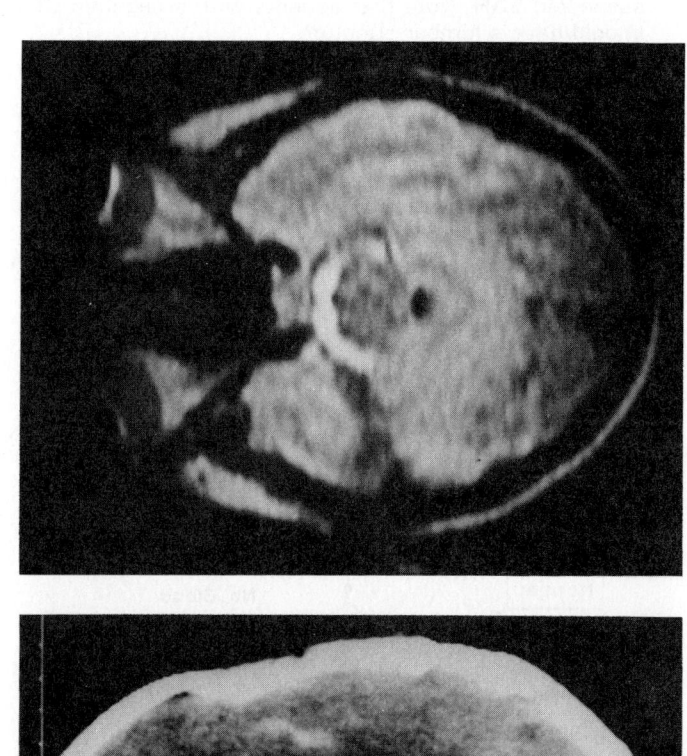

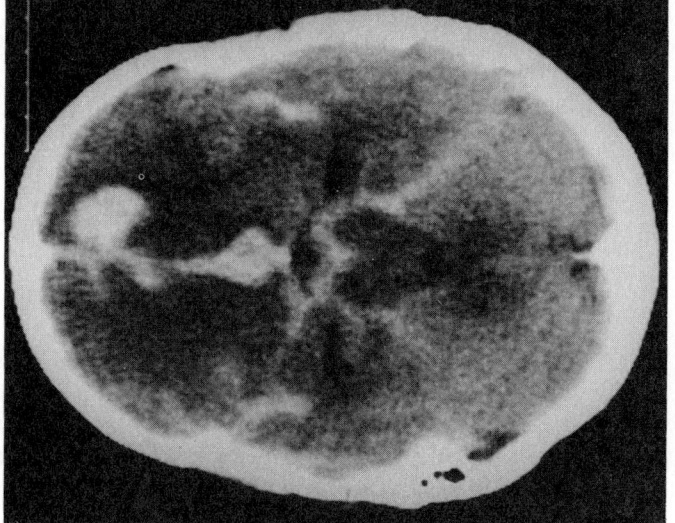

**Figure 4.1**: CT scan (left) and MR image (right) of patients with subarachnoid haemorrhage. The CT scan shows subarachnoid blood in the basal cisterns, and interhemispheric blood with a small right frontal intracerebral haematoma which suggests a ruptured anterior communicating artery aneurysm. Blood in the prepontine cistern is seen as white on the MR image.

**Figure 4.2:** Algorithm for management of patients with suspected SAH. Note that patients with a negative CT scan should have a lumbar puncture

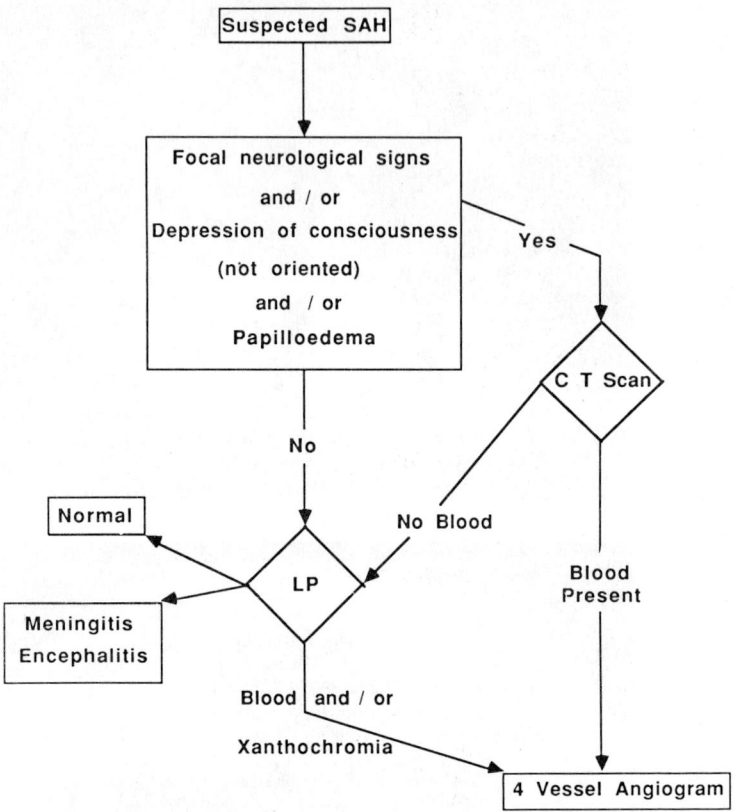

CT scanning which will help to define the site of haemorrhage, allow measurements of ventricular size and permit the exclusion of other causes such as tumour. The next step is a four-vessel angiogram which is best performed via the femoral route using a catheter under local anaesthesia. The *whole* intracranial circulation should be visualised because the management of a patient with multiple aneurysms may be different from that of a patient with a single aneurysm. Similarly, if an AVM is found, there may be an aneurysm on the arteries which supply it and this also demands a different approach. Angiography is usually performed at an early stage so that a decision on the timing of surgery can be taken with all the anatomical information available.

## 3. Subarachnoid haemorrhage of unknown aetiology

In some patients another cause for SAH such as a tumour or even a head injury may be found. If there is no cause of haemorrhage on four-vessel angiography, then the risk of further bleeding is negligible and the patient and family can be reassured.

## TREATMENT

Most patients with SAH are treated with bed rest, although evidence that this prevents rebleeding is lacking. However, if patients have lost autoregulation, then standing up may lead to a fall in MABP and, consequently, to a fall in CBF. Routine practice is therefore to keep these patients flat in bed.

## Care of the unconscious patient

A great number of patients who initially go into coma will rapidly recover and may regain full consciousness. Persistent coma is usually due to massive subarachnoid haemorrhage, intracerebral haemorrhage, subdural haemorrhage, acute hydrocephalus or ischaemic brain damage. The cause should be determined and treated appropriately. General management of the unconscious patient includes protection of the airway, attention to nutrition, maintenance of *normal* fluid and electrolyte balance, and care of the skin and eyes.

## Cardiovascular system

Many patients have reflex *hypertension* following their haemorrhage, and treatment of this may lead to a fall in CPP (especially if ICP is still elevated). It is probably safest *not* to reduce MABP acutely in these patients. With longstanding hypertension on the other hand, the treatment regime which controlled the hypertension prior to the haemorrhage should be maintained. Two additional cardiac abnormalities commonly occur. These are the reflex coronary artery spasm, which may produce *myocardial infarction*, and a wide variety of different *arrhythmias*, which may result from subendocardial infarction.

## Antifibrinolytic agents

These agents at first appeared attractive because it was thought that they should prevent the lysis of clots around the ruptured aneurysm. After preliminary enthusiasm for epsilon-aminocaproic acid and tranexamic acid it has become clear from a multi-centre prospective randomised placebo-controlled trial that, although these agents reduced the rebleed rate, they increased the incidence of ischaemic brain damage. The result was that the overall outcome was no better than with the use of a placebo. Current evidence therefore indicates that antifibrinolytic agents should *not* be used in patients with SAH.

## OPERATIVE TREATMENT

### 1. Aneurysms

The surest way to prevent rebleeding is to clip the aneurysm that has bled. In most patients with aneurysmal SAH, a single aneurysm is demonstrated and the only decision required is *when* to operate. In most series the operative mortality has been reduced to less than 10% and in some series, with delayed surgery, mortality is less than 1 or 2%. The problem with these delayed operations is that patients who are in good condition may rebleed and die during the waiting period. For this reason, early surgery would appear to be the best way to prevent rebleeding. Early surgery was once thought to be associated with a higher incidence of delayed cerebral ischaemia and therefore became unpopular. Over the last decade, more and more reports of successful operation within the first week of haemorrhage have appeared, with a surprisingly low mortality rate (Table 4.1). *It has become clear that it is safe to operate at any time if the patient is oriented and without focal neurological deficit. There is therefore little justification for delaying surgery in patients who are in good condition.*

The problem of surgery in patients who are confused or in coma or who have focal neurological signs has not been resolved. To make

**Table 4.1:** Type of management and final outcome in a series of 251 patients

| Outcome | Emergency operation | Early operation Grades I–III | Early operation Grades IV–V | Late operation | No operation | Total cases |
|---|---|---|---|---|---|---|
| Good recovery | 3 | 75 | 2 | 23 | 4 | 107 |
| Morbidity | 8 | 20 | 3 | 5 | 11 | 47 |
| Mortality | 8 (42%) | 4 (4%) | 1 (17%) | 1 (3%) | 83 (85%) | 97 (39%) |
| Total cases | 19 | 99 | 6 | 29 | 98 | 251 |

Source: from Ljunggren *et al.* (1985).

an impact on the disease of SAH, most clinicians have agreed that it is the *management mortality* which is important, and not the *operative mortality*. In other words, very late surgery with a low *operative mortality* may be associated with a high incidence of rebleeding in patients awaiting operation, and thus a high *management mortality*. To resolve this issue, an international co-operative study of the timing of aneurysm surgery has been undertaken and this has indicated that the *management mortality* with surgery planned within the first 3 days is better than with surgery planned at any other time for patients who are oriented and without focal neurological deficits. It therefore seems clear that patients in good condition following SAH should be investigated and their aneurysms clipped at the earliest opportunity. Nevertheless, those patients who have lost autoregulation of CBF are particularly sensitive to changes in MABP, so extreme care should be taken to maintain CPP at all times in their management. In particular, *hypotensive anaesthesia* (useful in patients with large aneurysms or in patients who have completely recovered from their initial bleed) should be avoided whenever *early surgery* is undertaken. If these patients should develop delayed cerebral ischaemia post-operatively, then hypervolaemic hypertensive treatment can be used to increase CBF by elevating the systolic blood pressure to about 180 mmHg.

*Multiple aneurysms*

These should be considered separately because only one of them will have bled, and only that aneurysm carries a high risk of rebleeding. All other aneurysms are regarded as unruptured, and each will carry a risk of haemorrhage of between 1 and 2% per annum. Two problems immediately present themselves:

(1) It may not be possible to decide which aneurysm has bled — clipping the wrong aneurysm may leave the patient exposed to a high risk of haemorrhage, added to the risk of craniotomy.
(2) If delayed post-operative ischaemia develops, then it is not safe to use hypervolaemic hypertensive treatment because it may *cause* haemorrhage from one of the unclipped aneurysms.

To decide which aneurysm has bled, the CT scan, or recently nuclear magnetic resonance imaging, may demonstrate the origin of the blood. If this is unhelpful, then the larger the aneurysm the greater the risk of haemorrhage. Clinical features, the electroencephalogram and the appearance of spasm on the angiogram may also act as guides as to which aneurysm has bled. However, in a proportion of patients, it is still impossible to decide and for this reasons surgeons have tended to favour the clipping of all accessible aneurysms through one craniotomy. If contralateral or inaccessible aneurysms are present, in addition to one that has bled, then early surgery should be avoided to minimise the risks of delayed cerebral ischaemia. Delaying surgery in this situation prevents the risk of haemorrhage that would be associated with hypervolaemic hypertensive treatment should it become necessary.

## Unruptured aneurysms

These either present themselves as incidental findings in patients undergoing angiography for other reasons, or they are diagnosed in association with a ruptured aneurysm. The incidence of haemorrhage for an unruptured aneurysm is between 1 and 2% per annum, so the age of the patient must be considered when evaluating the risk of rupture. A young person with a life expectancy of 50 years therefore has a high risk of haemorrhage during his or her lifetime. By contrast, an older patient, with a life expectancy of only 10 years, may prefer to avoid the risks of surgery.

## Giant aneurysms

These lesions present a special technical problem because of the difficulty in preserving the continuity of the parent vessels and branches when applying a large clip across what is often a wide neck. Previously, carotid ligation was recommended for giant intracranial aneurysms, but this procedure was associated with a significant rebleed rate and a risk of delayed stroke on long-term follow-up. More recently the combination of an extracranial/ intracranial arterial bypass together with an internal carotid artery ligation has been shown to be effective in treating giant aneurysms which cannot be clipped.

## Aneurysms associated with intracerebral haemorrhage

In patients with intracerebral haemorrhage due to an aneurysm, two problems present themselves:

(1) the necessity to remove the haematoma;
(2) the need to apply a clip as prophylaxis against further haemorrhage.

First, early removal of the haematoma does not improve the

patient's clinical condition or the outcome. Secondly, early clipping of the aneurysm in this situation may be dangerous. Surgery should therefore be delayed until the patient has started to make a recovery from the effects of the initial intracerebral haemorrhage. The clot should then be evacuated and the aneurysm clipped.

## 2. Arteriovenous malformations

Craniotomy and excision of an arteriovenous malformation is recommended when the lesion is accessible and when it is judged to be safe to remove it without producing a major neurological deficit. Advances in neuroradiology, embolisation techniques and the introduction of intraluminal balloon occluders, as well as intra-operative angiography, have made it possible to excise some lesions which were previously considered inoperable. A grading system has been described recently, and this helps to predict the morbidity of surgical excision (Table 4.2).

**Table 4.2:** Correlation of grade with surgical results (Spetzler and Martin, 1986)

|  | Minor deficit (%) | Major deficit (%) | Mortality (%) |
|---|---|---|---|
| Grade I | 0 | 0 | 0 |
| Grade II | 5 | 0 | 0 |
| Grade III | 12 | 4 | 0 |
| Grade IV | 20 | 7 | 0 |
| Grade V | 19 | 12 | 0 |

Grading is based upon size ($<$ 3 cm = 1; 3–6 cm = 2; $>$ 6 cm = 3) eloquence of adjacent brain (add 1 if eloquent) and venous drainage (add 1 if deep).

Small ($<$ 2cm) and inaccessible AVMs (e.g. brainstem, basal ganglia) can now be treated successfully with stereo-radiosurgery. Dural AVMs fed by the external carotid artery are probably best treated by intraluminal embolisation by an experienced neuroradiologist.

## CONCLUSIONS

The surgical results in patients with aneurysms have improved progressively over the last half-century. This was initially achieved by delaying surgery until the patient was in good clinical condition. However, these acceptable operative results were not matched by an improvement in the overall management mortality for SAH. Recent studies have shown that in patients in good clinical condition early surgery for single aneurysms can improve management mortality. Difficulty remains in patients who are not in good clinical condition, who have multiple or giant aneurysms or who have associated intracerebral haematomas. Whatever the clinical picture, the management of SAH has become a specialised field and *early referral* of patients in good clinical condition is essential if the overall outcome for the majority of patients is to be improved.

## FURTHER READING

Crompton, M.R. (1964) Infarction following the rupture of cerebral berry aneurysms. *Brain 87*, 263–9

Drake, C.G. (1981) Management of cerebral aneurysms. *Stroke 12*, 273–83

Kassell, N.F., Peerless, D.M., Durward, W.J. *et al.* (1982) Treatment of ischaemic deficits from vasospasm with intravascular volume expansion and induced arterial hypertension. *Neurosurgery 11*, 227–43

Ljunggren, B., Saveland, H., Brandt, L., *et al.* (1985) Early operation and overall outcome in aneurysmal subarachnoid haemorrhage. *J. Neurosurg. 62*, 547–51

Locksley, H. (1966) Natural history of subarachnoid haemorrhage, intracranial aneurysms and arteriovenous malformation. Section 5, Part 2. *J. Neurosurg. 25*, 321–68

Parkarinen, S. (1967) Incidence, etiology, and prognosis of primary subarachnoid haemorrhage. *Acta Neurol. Scand. 43* (Suppl.), 29

Sengupta, R. and McAllister, V.L. (1986) *Subarachnoid haemorrhage*, Springer-Verlag, Berlin

Spetzler, R.F. and Martin, N.A. (1986) A proposed grading system for arteriovenous malformation *J. Neurosurg. 65*, 476–83

Walker, A.E., Robins, M. and Weinfeld, F.D. (1981) National Survey of Stroke: clinical findings. *Stroke 12*, 113–31

Winn, H.R., Richardson, A.E. and Jane, J.A. (1977) The long term prognosis in untreated cerebral aneurysm: a ten year evaluation of 364 patients. *Ann. Neurol. 1*, 358–70

# 5

# Stroke

Peter Sandercock

## INTRODUCTION

Is stroke really an emergency? Certainly, many patients and their relatives regard a stroke as an emergency requiring immediate medical attention because of its dramatic onset and a feeling that a stroke, like a heart attack, is usually rapidly fatal. On the other hand, there are undoubtedly a few patients, generally with minor strokes, who may not seek medical help at all. Doctors' attitudes to stroke vary widely, though the majority probably do not regard stroke as an emergency mainly because they feel that 'nothing can be done'.

Community-based surveys suggest that only a small proportion of stroke patients are likely to benefit from urgent medical or surgical treatment. However, that is not to say that one can take a *laissez-faire* attitude to dealing with patients and their families. The general practitioner should ideally treat every stroke patient as a *potential* emergency in order to reduce the anxiety and concern of patients and their families and to identify as early as possible the patients likely to benefit from specialist referral or hospital admission.

New cases of stroke are relatively uncommon in general practice; the average general practitioner with a list size of 2000 can expect about four new cases of stroke each year. However, the differential diagnosis is wide and the GP may need to consider the diagnosis of stroke a good deal more often than that. The cornerstone of successful management of stroke in general practice is accurate diagnosis; careful clinical assessment is often much more helpful than expensive investigations.

## DEFINITIONS OF STROKE

The World Health Organization (WHO) definition of stroke is 'the rapid onset of signs of focal, and at times global (applied in cases in deep coma and with subarachnoid haemorrhage) loss of cerebral function, with symptoms lasting more than 24 hours or leading to death'. The definition is a clinical one and makes no assumptions about the underlying pathological type of stroke (cerebral infarction, primary intracerebral haemorrhage or subarachnoid haemorrhage). Though there are certain aspects of treatment and rehabilitation which are common to the management of all strokes, a knowledge of the pathological type of stroke can sometimes be vital for correct treatment.

## PATHOLOGICAL TYPES OF STROKE

### Cerebral infarction

Over 80% of all first strokes are due to cerebral infarction. It is becoming clear that there are at least two types of cerebral infarction syndrome: 'lacunar' infarction (Figure 5.1) when the neurological deficit is restricted and is due to occlusive thrombotic disease of a single small deep penetrating artery; and 'large' infarction (Figure 5.2) when the deficit is more extensive and is often due to embolic occlusion of larger vessel(s), such as the main trunk of the middle cerebral artery. The emboli come from either the heart (e.g. thrombus in the left atrium) or break off the surface of atheromatous plaques at the origin of the internal carotid artery. The natural history and prognosis of these two groups are different; patients with lacunar infarction have a lower case-fatality rate and better functional outcome. It is not yet clear though whether the investigation and treatment of these two subtypes of cerebral infarction need necessarily be different.

### Primary intracerebral haemorrhage

Although only 10% of first strokes are due to haemorrhage primarily into brain substance (Figure 5.3), it has become apparent, since the advent of CT scanning, that it is impossible reliably to distinguish primary intracerebral haemorrhage from cerebral

**Figure 5.1:** Lacunar infarction. The patient, a 60-year-old man, suddenly developed weakness of the right arm and leg. Speech and other cerebral function was normal and there was no sensory disturbance in the arm or leg. The CT scan shows a small infarct (arrow) in the left basal ganglia/internal capsule

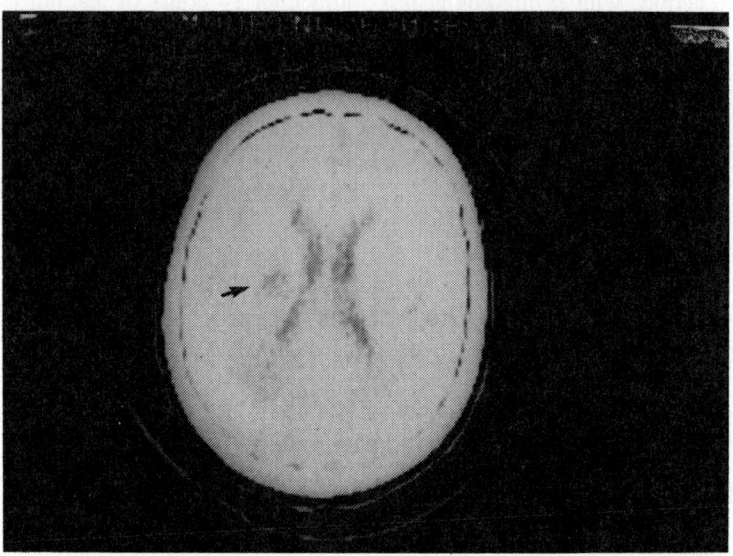

infarction on clinical grounds alone. In other words, if, for example, you want to treat a stroke patient with anticoagulants (or possible even aspirin), you must perform a CT scan to exclude haemorrhage before starting any treatment.

## Spontaneous subarachnoid haemorrhage (SAH)

Between 4 and 8% of all first strokes are due to subarachnoid haemmorhage. The commonest cause is rupture of a berry aneurysm and, less often, an arteriovenous malformation. When a patient presents to hospital with a clinical syndrome of sudden onset of severe headache, neck stiffness, vomiting and photophobia, the diagnosis is fairly straightforward. The diagnosis of SAH in general practice is often far from simple, as the following case demonstrates.

A 45-year-old man came home from work, and complained to his wife that he felt tired. After supper he suddenly developed a severe

**Figure 5.2:** Large infarction. This patient suddenly developed a hemiplegia with aphasia and a right homonymous hemianopia, indicating an extensive cerebral lesion. The CT scan correspondingly shows a large area of infarction (arrows) in the territory of the left middle cerebral artery

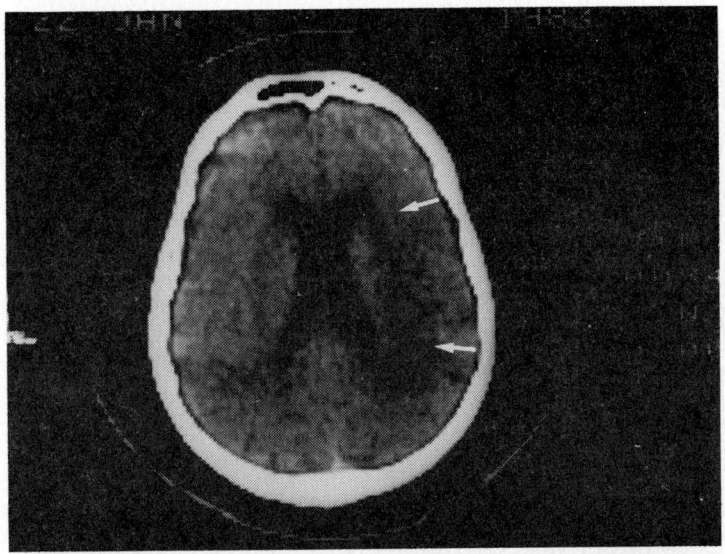

headache and vomited back his supper. He went to bed, and when the GP saw him an hour or so later he felt better though he still had a bad headache. On examination, there were no abnormal signs and there was no neck stiffness. The GP quite reasonably diagnosed migraine but visited again the next morning, by which time the patient was complaining of neck stiffness. The patient was admitted to hospital, where lumbar puncture and CT (Figure 5.4) confirmed a diagnosis of subarachnoid haemorrhage.

The main clue to the correct diagnosis was the suddenness of the onset of the headache; migraine usually evolves gradually over minutes or hours. Neck stiffness is not always present in the early stages of SAH, as the blood takes time to get down to the cervical subarachnoid space. Unfortunately, many patients with subarachnoid haemorrhages have 'warning leaks' which pass unrecognised, either because the patient or their doctor ignores them; this error can truly be said to be fatal, because the second bleed may often lead to death or severe disability.

**Figure 5.3:** Primary intracerebral haemorrhage. This 55-year-old carpenter suddenly lost the use of his arm and leg. The CT scan shows a small haemorrhage (arrow) in the basal ganglia. Clinically, his stroke was indistinguishable from that of the patient described in Figure 5.1

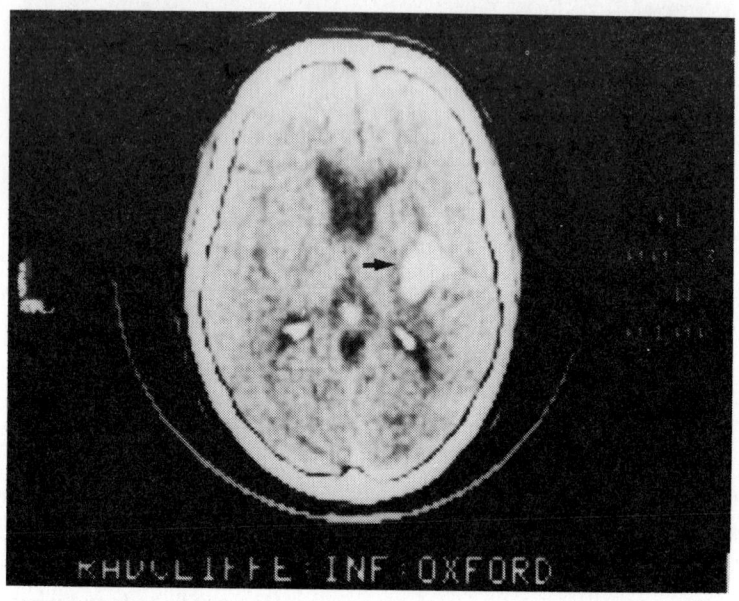

## CLINICAL DIAGNOSIS OF STROKE AND SOME COMMON STROKE SYNDROMES

### History of onset

Getting a clear history of the mode of onset (see Table 5.1) is the single most important item in sorting out a patient with a stroke. This is usually easier for the GP than the hospital doctor, since the patient's relatives will often be present at the time of the GP's visit to give further details of the mode of onset of the neurological deficit. The following case illustrates the problem.

A 70-year old lady was found lying on the floor by the night staff of the nursing home where she lived. She was unable to speak or to move the right arm and leg. The GP quite reasonably

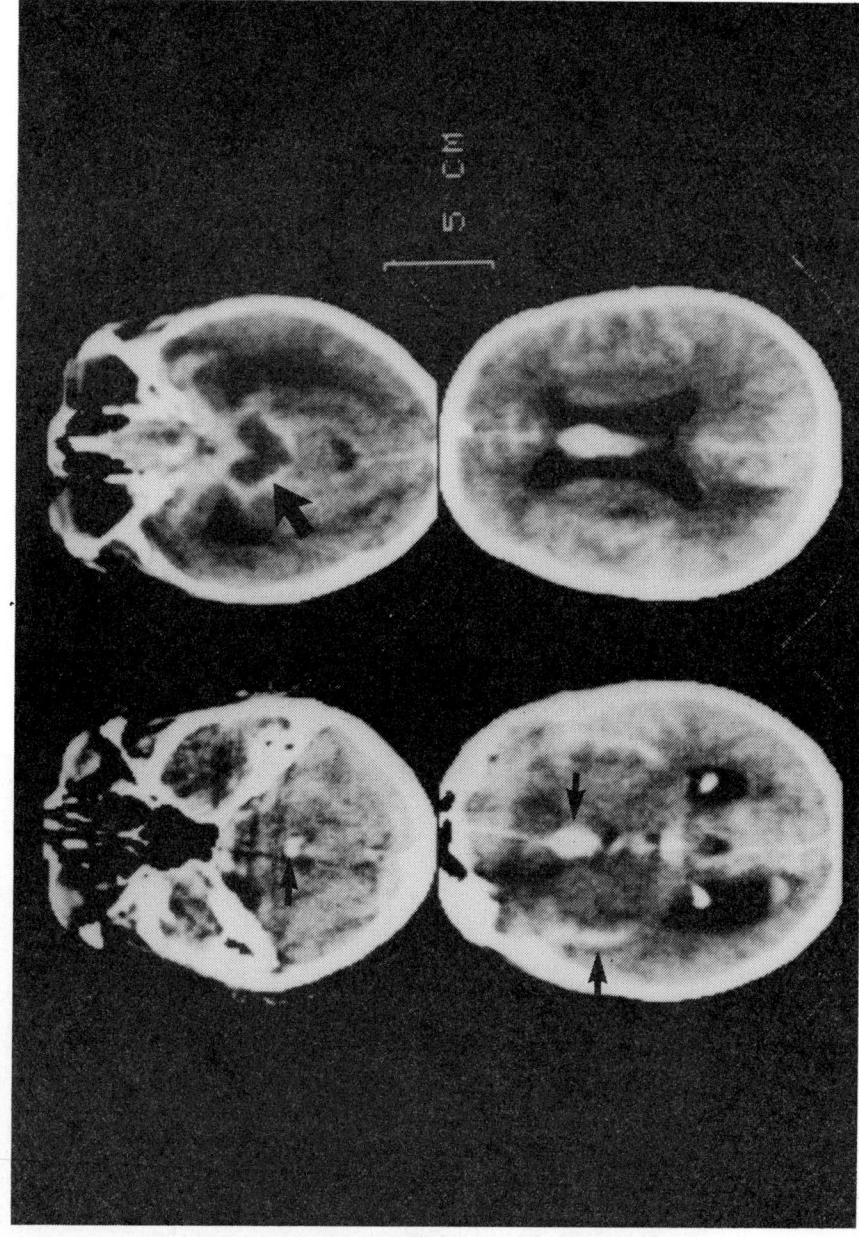

**Figure 5.4:** Spontaneous subarachnoid haemorrhage. Blood in the subarachnoid spaces shows up as lighter grey than the surrounding brain (arrows)

**Table 5.1:** Differential diagnosis in each stroke syndrome

*Sudden onset of focal neurological deficit*
Stroke
Cerebral tumour
Cerebral abscess
Subdural haematoma
Todd's paresis following focal epileptic seizure
Hypoglycaemia

*Sudden onset of coma, few or no focal signs and no meningism present*
Metabolic disturbance
   hypoglycaemia
   drug overdose
   hepatic, renal, endocrine failure
Post-ictal state
Cerebellar stroke with obstructive hydrocephalus[a]
Very early subarachnoid haemorrhage

*Sudden onset of coma with few or no focal signs and meningism present*
Subarachnoid haemorrhage
Meningitis

a. Acute cerebellar stroke may present this way, though there is usually time for the patient to develop symptoms and signs of cerebellar/brainstem dysfunction before becoming comatose.

**Figure 5.5:** CT scan showing left hemisphere malignant glioma (arrow) in a patient with slowly progressive dysphasia and weakness of the right arm

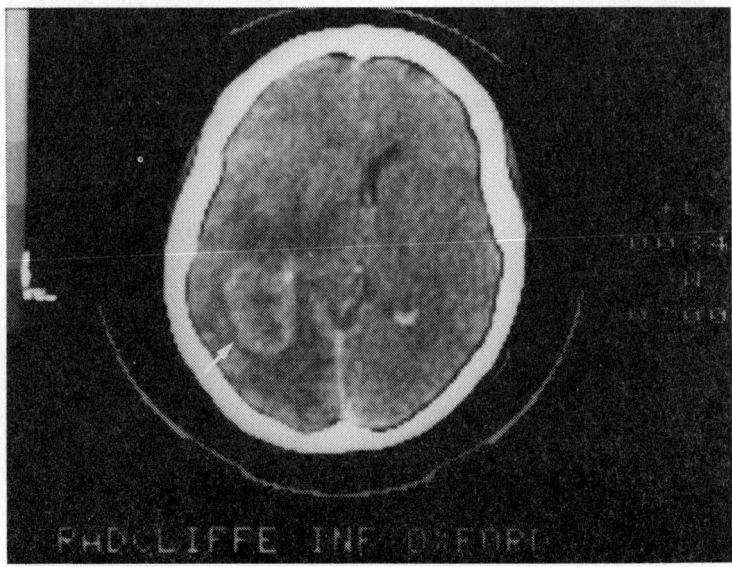

diagnosed a stroke. When he returned to see the patient the next day, he spoke to the matron of the home, who knew the patient well. She said the patient had had progressive difficulty finding words over the past few months, and more recently had difficulty using her right hand. With the additional information suggesting a much more gradual evolution of the deficit, the GP changed his diagnosis to cerebral tumour, and arranged a neurological consultation. The neurologist arranged a CT scan which showed a left-hemisphere glioma (Figure 5.5).

Since the patient could not give a history, the initial diagnosis had to be based on the information from the night staff and it seemed to indicate quite clearly that she had had a stroke. It was only with the information from the matron, suggestive of a slowly progressive left-hemisphere lesion, that the GP considered the correct diagnosis of cerebral tumour.

One should always be cautious about making a diagnosis of stroke where no clear history is available — usually because the patient is confused, drowsy or aphasic — and there is no witness to confirm the mode of onset. However, it often happens in hospital that the patient is unable to give a history and no relatives are available. The answer is simple; by making use of that extremely useful neurological instrument, the telephone, to obtain a clear history of a sudden onset, the hospital doctor will be able to make an accurate diagnosis of stroke *without* the need for CT scanning in the vast majority of cases.

## Focal symptoms and signs

The first hallmark of a stroke is its sudden onset. The second (except in cases of SAH) is the presence of focal symptoms and signs. When the focal sign happens to be a hemiparesis, the diagnosis of stroke may come to mind quite easily, though at least a quarter to a third of all strokes do not develop a hemiparesis. It is in the patients without a hemiparesis, who suddenly develop a more restricted deficit, that one may not immediately diagnose stroke: deficits such as aphasia alone, hemianopia alone, ataxia alone (usually misdiagnosed as 'labyrinthitis') and clumsiness of one hand (due to a small lesion in the cortex) all provide pitfalls even for the experts. Both of the following patients have had strokes.

A 75-year-old man was walking down to the post office. He stopped to cross the road and heard a car coming from the right, but could not see it until it had passed him. He thought at first that there was something wrong with his right eye, but then he realised that his left eye was affected too; he couldn't see anything to the right with either eye. The symptoms persisted. When examined at the neurology clinic a week later, the only deficit was a right homonymous hemianopia.

When a 55-year-old Polish welder working on a car assembly line, stopped for his tea break, he found that he was unable to unfasten the latch on his lunch box or grasp a match to light a cigarette. He was still able to hold his welding torch and to use it normally despite the problem with fine finger movements. On examination a few days later the only neurological abnormality was that he could not move the fingers of his right hand quickly or accurately. Despite the very limited neurological deficit, this was clearly a stroke, and since a CT scan was normal, his 'cortical hand' was probably due to a small infarct in the motor cortex. As in the previous case, the clue that this was a stroke was its sudden onset.

## Coma

It may be difficult to identify the cause of coma, particularly if no witness is readily available to give the history; this will often give important clues to the presence of a focal brain lesion, such as a history of hemiparesis, focal seizures and so on, or to some metabolic/toxic factor such as drug overdose. The examination of the unconscious patient is discussed elsewhere in this book, but is fairly straightforward; useful pointers to a *focal* brain lesion as the cause of the coma are asymmetry of either of the pupils, or the oculocephalic reflex (and/or caloric testing) or the response of the limbs to painful stimuli. In the absence of neuromuscular blocking agents such as curare or suxamethonium, an absent oculocephalic reflex almost always indicates a focal brain lesion as the cause of coma. In other words, a patient with asymmetrical pupils, who flexes his right arm and leg to pain but extends the left arm and leg to pain, is likely to have a focal lesion. Conversely, a patient with normal pupil reactions, normal oculocephalic reflexes and symmetrical limb responses to pain is likely to have a metabolic or toxic cause for their coma, such as drug overdose or hyper- or hypo-glycaemia.

Although careful examination is important, the history of the mode of the events around the time of the coma onset and other medical illnesses is the cornerstone of accurate diagnosis, as evidenced by the following.

A 75-year-old man was admitted via casualty with a provisional diagnosis of brainstem stroke. On examination he was hypertensive, drowsy, confused and had widely symmetrically dilated pupils and normal oculocephalic reflexes and flexed all four limbs equally to pain. The casualty officer had been unable to get a sensible history from the patient, so the medical registrar telephoned the patient's wife at home. She said that her husband had got up in the middle of the night with a troublesome cough, and had gone downstairs for some cough medicine. He returned a few minutes later, but gradually became confused and agitated over the next few hours. A search of the medicine cupboard revealed that he had taken embrocation by mistake. The pharmacist confirmed that the embrocation contained atropine. His symptoms were all compatible with atropine poisoning. He recovered over the next few days.

A 68-year-old lady with long-standing hypertension was admitted with a 'stroke'. Her sister said that she had been hypertensive for years, but had only been started on treatment one month previously. Shortly after starting she had had a similar 'stroke' in which she had become drowsy with no focal deficit. She had been admitted to a small hospital where she had recovered spontaneously. After discharge, she was restarted on her antihypertensives but had gradually become drowsy and confused over about 48 hours. There were no focal signs. Her serum sodium was 115 mmol/litre. After correction of hyponatraemia (presumably due to the diuretic), she recovered completely. Inquiry revealed her serum sodium after the first 'stroke' was 118 mmol/litre!

Both of these cases show how a careful clinical assessment with particular emphasis on the history, combined with simple laboratory tests, are often all that is required to make an accurate diagnosis in the unconscious patient. It is also important to keep an open mind about the diagnosis in patients with 'stroke'.

## Meningism

It is very important to test for meningism, though testing for it may be difficult when the patient is at home and in an awkwardly placed bed or chair. The presence of cervical osteoarthritis in the elderly may add further difficulties. None the less, any degree of meningism indicates either blood or infection in the subarachnoid space, and is always an indication for admission to hospital for lumbar puncture (LP). The contraindications to LP are given in Table 5.3 and are discussed in the section on investigation.

## Cerebellar stroke

This is a fairly uncommon stroke syndrome, but it is important because urgent surgical treatment may be life-saving. Swelling of the cerebellum because of infarction or haemorrhage can cause obstructive hydrocephalus by blocking the drainage of CSF through the fourth ventricle. In all but the most acute cases, the patient is alert at the onset and complains of brainstem or cerebellar symptoms (slurred speech, clumsiness, unsteadiness, double vision, hemi- or quadriparesis). As the lesion progresses and hydrocephalus develops, the patient's conscious level will in many cases then decline inexorably to death if the hydrocephalus is left untreated:

A 65-year-old man suddenly became dizzy and unsteady while walking his dog. His speech was slurred, and he was thought to be drunk. He fell to the ground and was taken to casualty. In casualty he was hypertensive with a blood pressure of 200/120 mmHg, and had dysarthria, nystagmus and a quadriparesis. The patient was admitted to the medical ward, where he gradually became more drowsy. Because the initial diagnosis was 'brainstem stroke', no action was deemed necessary. However, the medical senior house officer happened to mention the case to his neurological colleague over supper. The neurologist suggested the possibility of a cerebellar stroke, and a CT scan was arranged (Figure 5.6a) which showed obstructive hydro-cephalus. This was treated by ventricular drainage (Figure 5.6b) and the patient made a full recovery.

As with subarachnoid haemorrhage, the best way to avoid the pitfall is to consider the diagnosis more often, especially in stroke patients with 'brainstem stroke' and particularly if their conscious level is progressively declining.

## MANAGEMENT

### Admission to hospital

One of the most important management decisions for the GP or casualty officer is whether to admit the patient to hospital or not. Not all stroke patients need to be admitted, yet there are no widely accepted guidelines, as there are for head injury, for the selection of patients likely to benefit from admission.

*Do stroke patients fare better if admitted?*

There is marked variation around the world in the proportion of stroke cases occurring in the community who are admitted to hospital in the acute phase. In the Third World the proportion is not known but is probably small, whereas in some western countries the proportion may be as high as 80 or 90%. There are variations within countries too; in Britain, the percentage varies between 40 and 70%. We do not know whether a policy of admitting every stroke patient to hospital would improve outcome. Many patients with mild strokes make a complete recovery, and those with severe strokes often die rapidly irrespective of the treatment given, be it at home or in hospital. There is some evidence that patients with strokes of intermediate severity benefit from intensive rehabilitation. There is no clear evidence either for or against a policy of admitting all stroke patients to hospital. Many stroke patients prefer to stay at home; provided that the diagnosis of stroke is certain, that basic investigations have been performed and that social circumstances are adequate, it may be quite reasonable *not* to admit a patient.

*Medical factors weighing in favour of admission*

(a) *Doubt about the diagnosis.* Such doubt ('stroke' vs. 'not a stroke') often leads to admission for investigation. If GPs had access to a fast domiciliary or outpatient consultation service for acute stroke patients, the need for admission might be reduced.

(b) *Basic investigation.* Every patient with a stroke should have at least the investigations outlined in Table 5.2. All of these, with

83

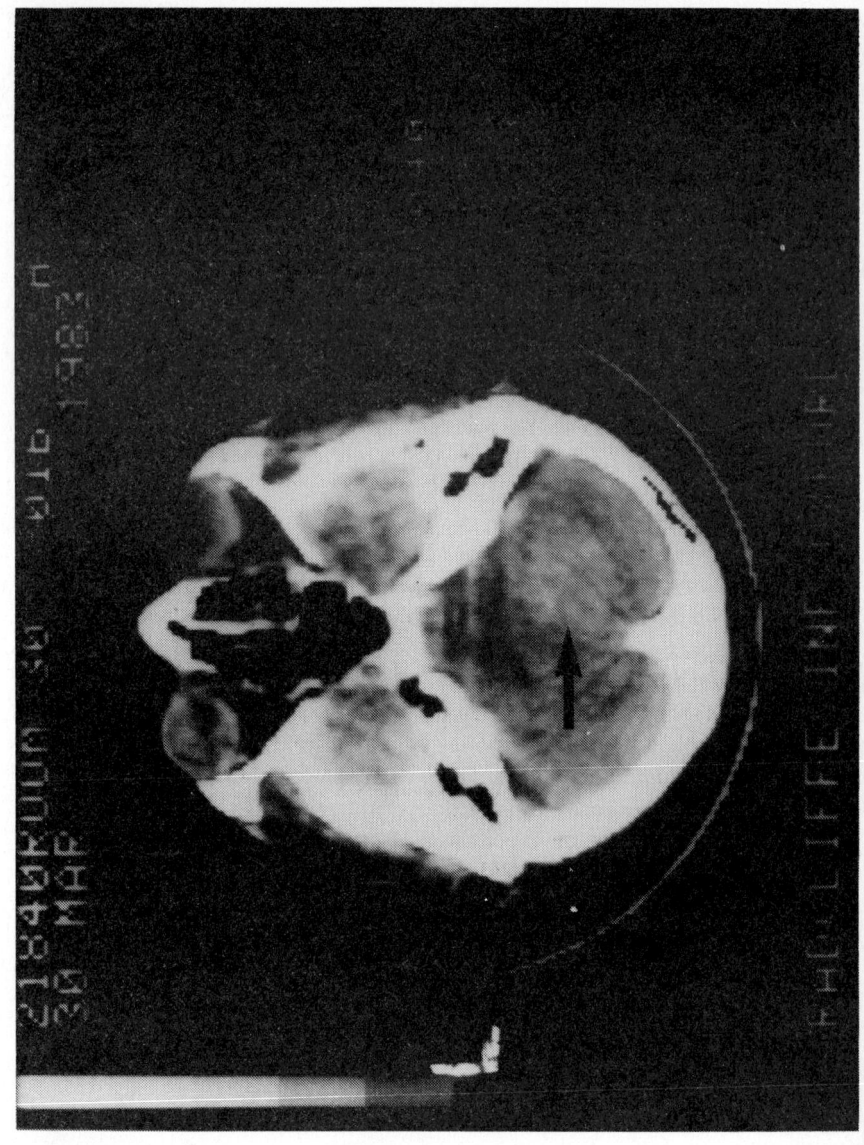

**Figure 5.6a:** Cerebellar stroke. A haematoma is visible in the cerebellar hemisphere (arrow) which has caused obstructive hydrocephalus and coma

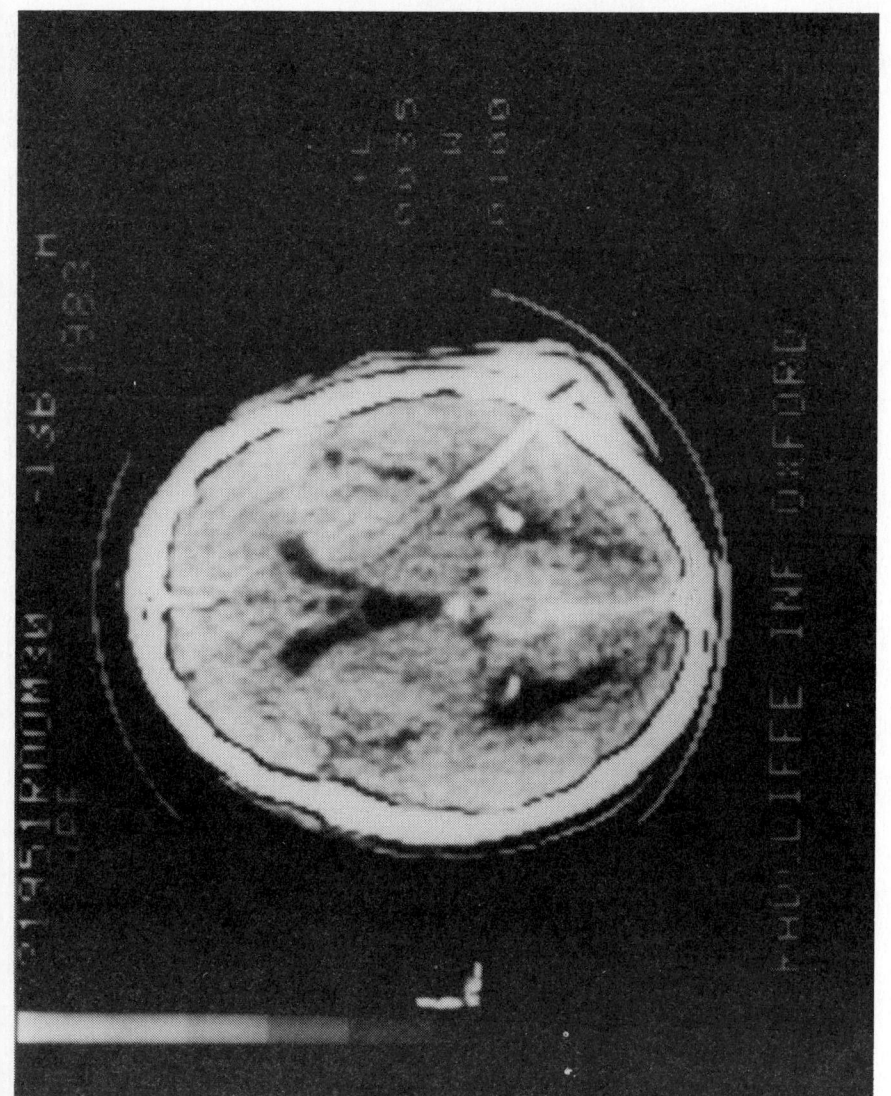

**Figure 5.6b:** CT scan after ventricular drainage. The drainage catheter can be seen. The ventricles have returned to near normal size

**Table 5.2**: Basic investigations for every patient with a stroke or TIA

| Test | Reason |
|---|---|
| Full blood count | Exclude polycythaemia, blood dyscrasia |
| Platelet count | Thrombocytosis/ thrombocytopaenia |
| Erythrocyte sedimentation rate (ESR) | Detect arteritis or subacute bacterial endocarditis (SBE) |
| Glucose | Diabetes is a risk factor. Hypo- and hyperglycaemia can cause focal neurological signs |
| Urea and electrolytes/biochemical profile | Metabolic disturbances mimic stroke |
| Serological tests for syphilis | Meningovascular syphilis is a rare but treatable cause of stroke |
| Chest X-ray | Assess any cardiac lesions. Unsuspected pneumonia |
| ECG | Detect ischaemic heart disease. Arrhythmia |

*Optional extras, depending on clinical features*

| | |
|---|---|
| Lipids | Young patient |
| Eosinophil count | Polyarteritis nodosa |
| Blood cultures | SBE |
| Autoantibody screen | Systemic lupus erythematosus (SLE) |
| Serum proteins and electrophoresis | Hyperviscosity syndrome |
| Sickle test in non-caucasians | Sickling |
| Urine homocysteine | Young stroke |
| Lumbar puncture | Meningism, syphilis |
| Temporal artery biopsy | Giant cell arteritis |
| Non-invasive ultrasound investigation of extracranial arteries | Selection for arteriography[a] |

[a] This test is not widely available in the UK.

the exception of the chest X-ray, can be arranged for patients at home or as an outpatient, and therefore the need for those tests should not of itself require admission.

(c) *Special investigations*. Lumbar puncture, CT scanning and cerebral arterial angiography are the most important investigations to consider. Lumbar puncture is indicated if there is a suspicion of SAH or meningitis. It should *not* be performed if there are focal neurological signs (such as hemiparesis, aphasia, cranial nerve palsies or marked asymmetry of the pupils) or

**Table 5.3:** Contraindications to lumbar puncture

(a) *A history of focal neurological symptoms*
Focal neurological deficit
  Hemiparesis
  Dysphasia
  Visuospatial disorder
  Hemianopia
  Oculomotor nerve palsy (III, IV, VI)
Seizures, especially if focal, or generalised with focal onset
  Motor
  Sensory
  Temporal lobe

(b) *Focal neurological signs*
In the conscious patient, as above
In the comatose patient
  Asymmetrical pupils/pupillary light response
  Asymmetrical oculocephalic reflex
  Absent oculocephalic reflex[a]/absent pupillary light responses
  Asymmetrical limb response to pain

(c) *Symptoms or signs of raised intracranial pressure*
Progressive headache of *recent* onset
  Exacerbated by bending/coughing
  Associated with transient postural visual obscurations
  Present on waking *and* improving soon after rising
Papilloedema[b]

[a] Provided no neuromuscular blocking agent present.
[b] The absence of papilloedema does not exclude raised intracranial pressure.
DO NOT USE MYDRIATICS IN AN UNCONSCIOUS PATIENT IN ORDER TO OBTAIN A BETTER VIEW OF THE OPTIC FUNDUS

symptoms or signs of raised intracranial pressure (Table 5.3). One should not use mydriatics in order to obtain a better view of the optic fundus, as pupillary size is one of the few useful neurological signs in an unconscious patient; in any case the absence of papilloedema does not rule out an intracranial mass lesion.

A CT scan is no substitute for a careful clinical assessment; a clear history of a sudden onset and the presence of appropriate focal neurological signs can lead to a confident and reliable diagnosis of stroke. The CT scan *cannot* make a diagnosis of stroke, not least because it may be normal in perhaps 30–50% of cerebral infarcts, a small proportion of primary intracerebral haemorrhages (especially if performed more than 3 weeks after the onset) and in milder cases of SAH. Similarly, cerebral infarcts and haemorrhages may, depending on the stage of their evolution at the time of the scan, appear identical to cerebral tumours and other pathology. In these cases, correct interpretation will depend on the history of the mode of onset of the deficit.

A 55-year-old widow, who lived alone, was admitted to hospital with a right hemiparesis and aphasia. CT scan showed an enhancing dominant hemisphere lesion which was reported as a glioma. Surgical biopsy was not performed, because of the lesion site. She was treated with dexamethasone and transferred to a nursing home for terminal care. Twelve months later, she was still alive, her speech better, but she was Cushingoid, with steroid myopathy and contractures of her right arm and leg. Physiotherapy had been deemed inappropriate because of her presumed very poor prognosis. Repeat CT scan showed a large left hemisphere infarct and not a tumour. This patient's disastrous clinical outcome might have been avoided if the CT scan findings had been interpreted in the light of the clinical details.

None the less, in an ideal world, a CT scan would be a helpful investigation in many patients with stroke, but is only likely to make an important difference to management in perhaps a third of all cases. The patients most likely to benefit from CT are listed in Table 5.4. Young patients aged under 40 with stroke are rare and merit CT scanning in their own right. Isotope brain scanning, available in many district general hospitals, like CT although often positive in cerebral infarction may often mistake infarction for a cerebral tumour; this may lead to inappropriate treatment.

The indications for cerebral angiography are given in Table 5.5. It is rarely performed in the acute phase of stroke or TIA but when the patient has made a complete or at least partial recovery, with the aim of identifying patients with internal carotid artery atheroma likely to benefit from carotid endarterectomy. The timing of angiography after SAH depends on the clinical conditions of the patient, but may be done as early as 24 hours after the bleed or as late as one week.

### Social factors

These are often the most important factors in determining whether a patient is admitted to hospital or stays at home. A caring family or neighbours, a suitable house with downstairs lavatory and/or

**Table 5.4:** Indications for CT scanning

*Doubt about the diagnosis of stroke*
Slowly progressive deficit (Figure 5.7)
No clear history obtainable because of coma, dysphasia or confusion
No clear focal signs

*Need to exclude intracranial haemorrhage*
Need to give/already on anticoagulants

(a)   Definite cardiac embolic source
      Artrial fibrillation *and* rheumatic heart disease
      Prosthetic heart valve
(b)   Pulmonary embolism/deep venous thrombosis

Need to give/already on antiplatelet agents
Candidate for carotid endarterectomy

*Suspected cerebellar stroke (Figures 5.5 and 5.6)*
Brain-stem/cerebellar symptoms and signs *and* decreasing conscious level
Sudden onset deep coma *and* no focal signs *and* no meningism *and* no metabolic disturbance

*Subarachnoid haemorrhage (Figure 5.4)*
Confirm the diagnosis
Identify which of multiple aneurysms has bled
Localise any haematoma
Identify cause for any deterioration after initial bleed (i.e. rebleed, vasospasm, hydrocephalus)

*Young stroke (aged < 40)*

bathroom and readily available day or night nursing support as appropriate are all factors which make it easier to cope with a patient at home. Concern on the part of the family, that 'something must be done' may lead to inappropriate admission to hospital; domiciliary assessment by a specialist may help to allay the anxiety that sometimes lies behind such attitudes.

## GENERAL MANAGEMENT OF THE ACUTE STROKE PATIENT

The first principle of management is to exclude treatable causes of stroke (Table 5.6). Almost all of these can be identified by a careful clinical assessment and the few simple tests outlined in Table 5.2.

**Table 5.5**: Indications for cerebral angiography

*Ischaemic stroke[a]*
Suitable for carotid endarterectomy, i.e. if all are true
  TIA or mild stroke with good recovery
  CT scan excludes intracerebral haemorrhage
  Event definitely in carotid artery territory
  Fit for surgery

Suspected non-atheromatous arterial disease
  Young stroke
  Arteritis[b]
  Arterial dissection[c]
  Stroke in a young patient with no causative factors[d]

*Haemorrhagic stroke*
Subarachnoid haemorrhage, i.e. if all are true
  Fit for surgery
  Not comatose
  Focal neurological deficit absent or minimal
  Primary bleeding disorder excluded

Primary intracerebral haemorrhage, i.e. if all are true
  Primary intracerebral haemorrhage confirmed by CT
  Primary bleeding disorder excluded
  Patient not hypertensive or haematoma not in a site normally
    associated with hypertensive bleeds

[a] Cerebral angiography is only rarely indicated in the acute phase of ischaemic stroke or TIA. It is normally performed once the patient has made a partial or complete recovery.
[b] If diagnosis cannot be established any other way.
[c] Often young strokes; may have a history of relatively minor neck injury.
[d] If no vascular risk factors such as hypertension, diabetes, and no cardiac source of embolism.

The second is to prevent the complications of stroke such as pressure sores, venous thrombo-embolism, pneumonia and frozen shoulder.

The third is to identify and treat vascular risk factors: hypertension, diabetes, hyperlipidaemia and smoking. This should also include a search for, and treatment of, manifestations of atheromatous vascular disease elsewhere: angina, myocardial infarction, abdominal aneurysms and intermittent claudication.

**Table 5.6:** Some important treatable causes of stroke

---

*Ischaemic stroke*
Arteritis
  Giant cell arteritis
  Systemic lupus erythematosus
  Polyarteritis nodosa
  Granulomatous angiitis
Blood disorders
  Polycythaemia
  Thrombocythaemia
Cardiac lesions causing emboli to brain
  Atrial fibrillation with rheumatic heart disease
  Extensive acute MI
  Artificial valve prostheses
  Subacute bacterial endocarditis (SBE)

*Haemorrhagic stroke*
Arteritis
Aneurysm
Arteriovenous malformation
Haemostatic defects
  Iatrogenic (warfarin overdosage)
  Thrombocytopaenia
  Inherited (haemophilia)

---

## Risk factor management

'Risk' factors can be divided into two kinds: factors that increase the risk of atheromatous arterial disease (by far the most important is hypertension, with diabetes mellitus, smoking and hyperlipidaemia less important), and clinical manifestations of atheromatous arterial disease outside the brain (angina, myocardial infarction, abdominal aneurysms and intermittent claudication).

### Treatment of hypertension in the acute phase of stroke or SAH

Hypertension is undoubtedly the single most important risk factor for both ischaemic and haemorrhagic stroke. In stroke-free patients, treatment of moderate to severe hypertension is likely to reduce the risk of stroke, perhaps by as much as 50%. We do not know whether the risk reduction is so great in patients who have had a stroke, but, clearly, close monitoring and appropriate treatment of raised blood pressure in the long term are likely to reduce the risk of further stroke.

*(a) When to treat after a stroke.* Blood pressures are often markedly elevated above their pre-stroke levels in the acute phase of stroke. They can be particularly high after subarachnoid haemorrhage. However, blood pressure will fall steadily over the week after the onset without any treatment, so a decision on treatment should be deferred unless there is clear retinal, renal or pulmonary evidence (i.e. pulmonary oedema) of accelerated hypertension. There is always a great temptation to 'do something' and to give antihypertensive agents within the first few hours of admission, in the belief that lowering blood pressure will prevent extension of the infarction or prevent further bleeding. It appears that quite the reverse is true. There is an area of critically perfused tissue around a fresh cerebral infarction — the so-called 'ischaemic penumbra' — which is potentially viable provided perfusion is maintained; lowering the perfusion pressure by injudicious antihypertensive therapy could theoretically increase the area of infarction and worsen the neurological deficit. In patients with SAH, who may have secondary vasospasm, the high arterial BP may be necessary to maintain cerebral perfusion.

However, blood pressures rise after discharge from hospital to pre-stroke levels. So, although a conservative approach to the management of hypertension is important in the early stages, blood pressures must be checked regularly after discharge from hospital, and treatment must be started and continued as appropriate. The GP is by far the best person to undertake the long-term management of risk factors, particularly hypertension, after stroke.

*(b) Which antihypertensive?* Unfortunately, intravenous and intramuscular hypotensive agents are still over-used in patients with acute stroke, sometimes with disastrous effects for the reasons described above. Oral antihypertensives given in the acute phase probably carry a similar but much smaller risk of deterioration.

The conclusion, then, is that, if at all possible, previously undetected arterial hypertension should be monitored closely for several days after a stroke. If it is sustained, oral agents should be used; intravenous agents are needed only rarely. Blood pressures *must* be checked after discharge from hospital.

*Other risk factors*

Diabetes mellitus needs treating in its own right. Treating hyperlipidaemia after stroke may produce a worthwhile reduction in the risk of *cardio*vascular events, but a less certain reduction in the risk of *cerebro*vascular events; younger patients with more to lose from a cardiac event might be advised on diets whereas no action would probably be necessary for older patients. Stopping cigarette smoking will likewise produce a worthwhile reduction in the risk of *cardio*vascular events, but a less certain reduction in the risk of *cerebro*vascular events; young patients should certainly be advised to stop.

*Manifestations of atheromatous vascular disease elsewhere*

Since cardiac events are more frequent than cerebral events after stroke, careful attention to the detection and treatment of angina and other forms of ischaemic heart disease may do more to improve the patient's outcome after stroke and TIA than some of the more attractive procedures such as carotid endarterectomy (see below).

## SPECIFIC TREATMENTS OFTEN USED (AND ABUSED) IN THE ACUTE PHASE

### Brain shrinking agents

Agents such as mannitol, glycerol and dexamethasone are of no value in the routine treatment of acute stroke. Dexamethasone may be used in the rare instance of a patient with CT-proven cerebellar stroke and secondary obstructive hydrocephalus admitted to a hospital with intensive neurological monitoring facilities, where surgical treatment can follow immediately if medical therapy fails.

### Calcium entry blockers

These appear to be promising agents, but more trials are needed and there is therefore no indication for giving them on a large scale as yet.

### Isovolaemic haemodilution in ischaemic stroke

Reduction of the haematocrit increases cerebral blood flow and cerebral oxygen delivery. Haemodilution by a combination of venesection and simultaneous volume replacement with low molecular weight dextran to prevent hypotension is a theoretically attractive treatment for acute ischaemic stroke and trials are in progress.

## PREVENTING RECURRENT CEREBRAL AND CARDIAC EVENTS IN THE LONG TERM

### Aspirin

The best evidence available suggests that regular aspirin in doses between 300 mg and 1 g daily reduces the risk of myocardial infarction, vascular death and stroke after TIA and minor ischaemic stroke. The risk of non-fatal myocardial infarction or non-fatal stroke is reduced by about 25% and the risk of vascular death by about 10%. It is therefore reasonable to give patients with TIA and minor stroke 300 mg daily, though the dose can be reduced to 75 mg if gastric side effects are troublesome. Small doses (30–75 mg) are the subject of current trials. The value of aspirin in patients with major stroke is not clear. Aspirin increases the risk of cerebral haemorrhage, but it is not clear whether every patient should have a CT scan to exclude haemorrhage before starting aspirin therapy.

### Other antiplatelet agents

The evidence on the value of the other antiplatelet agents — dipyridamole (Persantin), sulphinpyrazone (Anturan), ticlopidine and suloctidil — is scanty and statistically less reliable than the data on aspirin. Furthermore, aspirin has the dual advantages of being very much cheaper, and has a much better documented safety record than these newer agents. These agents therefore should not be used after stroke and TIA.

### Beta blockers

After the acute phase of the stroke, coronary heart disease is the commonest cause of death. Beta blockers reduce the risk of death and reinfarction in the months and years after a myocardial infarct. Since 25% of patients with a first stroke have some form of coronary heart disease, beta blockers would appear a promising treatment. Trials are in progress.

## Anticoagulants

There is no convincing evidence that anticoagulants reduce the risk of recurrent stroke in patients with cerebral infarction due to thrombo-embolism from atheromatous arterial disease. Anticoagulants may be of use in the few patients with cardiac lesions which carry a very high risk of embolisation: rheumatic heart disease (RHD) with atrial fibrillation (AF), and aortic or mitral artificial valve prosthesis (though probably not xeno- or homo-graft valve). There is no convincing evidence either for or against the use of anticoagulants in patients with AF but no RHD.

In the few patients with stroke in whom anticoagulants really are considered necessary, three points are important:

(1) *CT scan every patient before starting anticoagulants.* It is impossible to rule out intracerebral haemorrhage by clinical methods (Figure 5.7). Likewise, lumbar puncture is usually normal in patients with small intracerebral haemorrhages. The only reliable way to rule out intracerebral haemorrhage is by CT scanning. Thus every patient who is to be started on anticoagulants *must* have a CT scan before treatment is begun.

(2) *Contraindications.* Patients who have a severe neurological deficit, or a large area of infarction on the CT scan, or are hypertensive or elderly, or have any evidence of bacterial endocarditis should *not* be anticoagulated. In the absence of these contraindications it may be possible to start anticoagulants, but the risks of the cerebral infarct becoming haemorrhagic are still significant.

## Carotid endarterectomy

This operation removes atheromatous plaque from the origin of the internal carotid artery to try to prevent thrombi forming on the pathological surface and embolising to the cerebral circulation. If the operation is performed in the early stage after a stroke, there is an unacceptably high risk of further stroke and death, so it is normally performed once the patient has made a full, or at least substantial, recovery. However, we do not know if the operation really does reduce the risk of stroke, and if so, whether the risk reduction is offset by the operative mortality/serious morbidity rate of around 2–8%. The operation is only applicable to a relatively small proportion

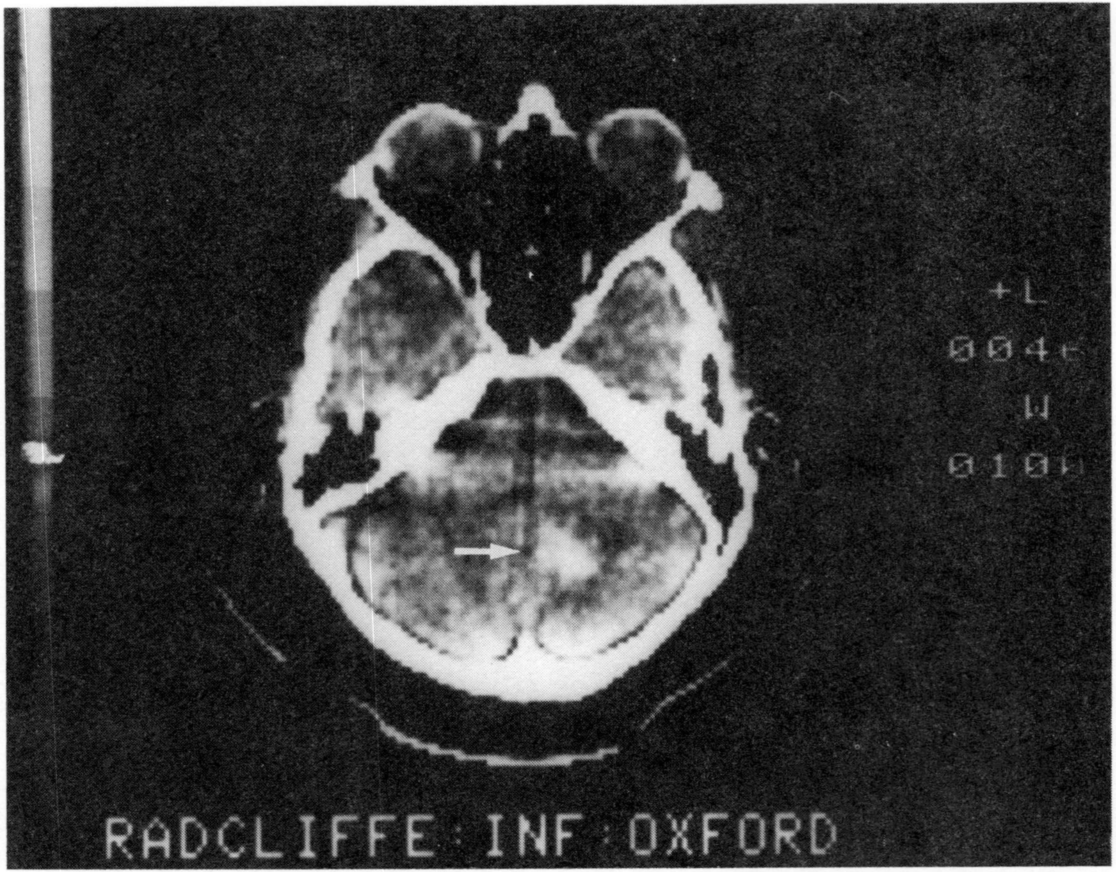

**Figure 5.7:** This 65-year-old patient suddenly became dizzy while standing at the sink. She had slurred speech and was unsteady when she walked. She had atrial fibrillation, but no valvular heart disease. The CT shows a small haematoma in the cerebellum (arrow). The general practitioner was going to start the patient on anticoagulants. Fortunately the CT scan result became available before anticoagulants were started

of patients with TIA and an even smaller proportion of patients with stroke. Table 5.5 lists the criteria for selecting patients for the operation. Multicentre trials of the value of the operation are in progress.

## Superficial temporal–middle cerebral artery bypass

This elegant operation fashions a bypass around surgically inaccessible stenosis of the internal carotid and/or middle cerebral artery (MCA). The superficial temporal artery is dissected and passed through a small craniotomy and anastomosed with a cortical branch of the MCA. A recent controlled trial has shown that it does not reduce the risk of stroke or death. The operation therefore has no part to play in either the acute or long-term management of patients with stroke or TIA.

## TALKING TO THE PATIENT AND THE RELATIVES

A stroke is often a frightening and bewildering experience for both the patient and the family. Inappropriate fear of impending death or lifelong disability may be compounded by difficulty in formulating or articulating speech and misinterpretation of what people are saying. Stressing the benign outcome after first stroke is important: data from the Oxfordshire Community Stroke Project clearly show that the prognosis for first stroke is not nearly as bad as is popularly believed (Table 5.7). At one year, about 30% will have died and 20% will be dependent, but the remaining 50% will be alive and independent in activities of daily living.

## CONCLUSION

Stroke certainly is an emergency from the point of view of the patient, the family and the GP. A small proportion of patients, who can be identified by bedside assessment and simple investigations, are truly neurological emergencies likely to benefit from urgent treatment. However, over-zealous use of some treatments, such as anticoagulants, antihypertensives and carotid surgery in the acute phase of stroke, can all be very hazardous to the patient. In the longer term, careful control of risk factors — especially hypertension — in all patients and regular aspirin use in patients with TIA

**Table 5.7:** Death or recurrence after first-ever stroke[a]

|  | Death (%) | | Recurrence |
| --- | --- | --- | --- |
|  | Acute (1) | 1 year (2) | (3) |
| All strokes | 20 | 32 | 11 |
| Cerebral infarction | 11 | 15 | 13 |
| Primary intracerebral haemorrhage | 56 | 19 | 6 |
| Subarachnoid haemorrhage | 43 | 6 | 4 |

(1) 30-day case fatality rate.
(2) 1-year case fatality rate in patients who survived at least one month after stroke.
(3) Proportion of patients who survived at least one month from stroke who suffered a recurrence in the next year.
[a] Data from the Oxfordshire Community Stroke Project.

and minor ischaemic stroke are of proven benefit in reducing the risk of recurrent stroke, heart attacks and vascular death. Beta blockers appear to be promising agents.

## SUMMARY

The *clinical* diagnosis of stroke is reliable provided a clear history of a sudden onset of a focal neurological deficit can be obtained. It may be unreliable if no clear history is obtainable, if consciousness is impaired, if meningism is present, if seizures have occurred, or if there are no clear focal signs.

Every patient with a first stroke should, at some stage in the acute illness, have a careful clinical assessment by a specialist and a few simple investigations. Basic investigation of stroke can be done in the home, so not all patients need admission to hospital. Patients likely to benefit from CT scanning and other investigations can be identified by simple clinical criteria.

Some patients with stroke require treatment (e.g. those with arteritis, bacterial endocarditis, cerebellar stroke). There is no single drug treatment that is of proven benefit in all patients with acute stroke.

Consistent application of basic nursing skills and simple physical treatments (e.g. support for the paretic arm by means of a pillow to prevent frozen shoulder) will avoid many of the complications of immobility after stroke. This basic principle is all too often neglected.

Most strokes are due to the thrombo-embolic complications of atheroma, so it is important in the long term to prevent not only recurrent stroke but also myocardial infarction and other serious vascular events, by careful assessment and treatment of vascular risk factors, treatment of ischaemic heart disease and the use of regular aspirin.

## FURTHER READING

Allen, C.M.C., Anderson, R., Bamford, J.M., Howse, A., Muir, J., Sandercock, P.A.G., Wade, D.T. and Warlow, C.P. (1986) *Stroke*, MTP Press, Lancaster

Harrison, M.J.G. and Dyken, M.L. (eds) (1983) *Cerebral Vascular Disease*, Butterworths, London

Ross Russell, R.W. (ed.) (1983) *Vascular diseases of the central nervous system*, Churchill Livingstone, Edinburgh

Sandercock, P.A.G., Molyneux, A.J. and Warlow, C.P. (1985) Value of computed tomography in patients with stroke: Oxfordshire Community Stroke Project. *Brit. Med. J. 290*, 193–7

Wade, D., Hewer, R.L., Skilbeck, C.F. and David, R.M. (1985) *Stroke: a critical approach to diagnosis, treatment and management*, Chapman & Hall, London

Warlow, C.P. and Morris, P.J. (eds) (1982) *Transient Ischaemic Attacks*, Marcel Dekker, New York

# 6

## Epilepsy

### John Patten

**INTRODUCTION**

As stressed in Chapter 1 the direct requirement for skilled management of acute medical conditions is accurate diagnosis and recognition of the emergent nature of the situation. This is particularly true in the field of impaired, altered or complete loss of consciousness, which is one of the most frequent causes of acute admission to the neurological unit. As discussed below, in few instances is immediate admission and urgent treatment actually necessary. It is usually the anxiety of the patient, their relatives or their medical advisors that prompts such attention. In the vast majority of cases no serious underlying disease will be identified and alarm is unnecessary. Prompt identification of the seizure type and knowledge of the likely outcome will govern the speed and nature of supportive care and anticonvulsant treatment.

Epileptologists have attempted complex classifications of the epilepsies to standardise the reporting of events and the reporting of clinical trials. There is also the hope that clearer classification will rationalise therapy. The latest revision of the international classification of seizures recognises three major groupings.

(1) Focal (partial, local) seizures are classified in three subgroups, simple focal seizures, complex focal seizures and focal seizures evolving to generalised tonic, clonic convulsions. Further subdivisions of these groupings result in no less than 27 subtypes to cover all aspects of focal phenomenology and variable degrees of altered consciousness. This includes what was previously called temporal lobe or psychomotor epilepsy and is now classified as complex partial seizures.

(2) Generalised (convulsive or non-convulsive) seizures are divided into six major groupings and nine subgroups which include what was formerly called petit mal and grand mal.

(3) Unclassified seizures: where inadequate data preclude accurate identification, and unusual episodes, particularly in neonates, where certainty as to their epileptic nature remains in doubt.

Status elipepticus is the term used when any form of seizure persists or is repeated sufficiently frequently that recovery between attacks does not occur or an attack lasts longer than 30 minutes, There is evidence that brain damage is caused by attacks lasting over 20 minutes. Continuing focal (Jacksonian) epilepsy, when very localised, is referred to as epilepsia partialis continua. In the generalised epilepsies both absence status and tonic–clonic status occur, the latter being the most serious and life-threatening complication of epilepsy.

In spite of the attempts to re-define epilepsy, for practical considerations and relative simplicity I propose to discuss the recognition, complications and treatment of epilepsy under major headings only, using time-honoured terminology. Febrile convulsions are discussed in detail as such episodes represent an important group in general practice. Other varieties of epilepsy such as akinetic grand mal, the myoclonic epilepsies and rare variants of incomplete seizures can present both diagnostic and treatment problems. Further coverage of these conditions is beyond the scope of the present chapter. The discussion is primarily aimed at the correct identification and diagnostic and treatment pitfalls of the common epilepsies.

## GENERAL OBSERVATIONS AND PRINCIPLES

For practical purposes, whatever the subsequent phenomena, the onset of the epileptic attack is instantaneous, as if a switch had been thrown. The recognition of this abruptness is probably the single most important feature raising the suspicion of epilepsy. The recovery period is often less well defined especially in those cases where consciousness has been impaired. Where consciousness is unimpaired, the diagnosis can often be made from the patient's own observations. In some cases of complex partial seizures (temporal lobe or psychomotor epilepsy), the patient may have a very distorted perception of the duration of the event and his or her behaviour

101

during the attack. In this group, additional eye-witness observations can be quite invaluable and sufferers are often amazed at revelations of which they have no knowledge. Where unconsciousness occurs, or the patient is only aware of coming to on the floor, eye-witness accounts provide the only useful diagnostic information. The use of the EEG as a diagnostic tool and final arbiter in suspected epilepsy is flawed by the deficiencies of the technique and the variability of epileptic activity in the EEG. The value and appearance of the EEG in the different types of epilepsy is discussed below. The treatment of the acute attack is governed by the seizure type, and subsequent prophylactic therapy by the patient's response to medication. This may in some instances lead to reconsideration of the diagnosis or the seizure type. In general some response to treatment, however unimpressive, is seen, and the total failure of medication, when serum levels have established compliance and adequate dosage, should prompt immediate reappraisal of the diagnosis.

## FEBRILE CONVULSIONS

Febrile convulsions are reported to occur in 2–8% of children under the age of 6. By definition, the patient will be a child, usually aged between 18 months and 6 years. Such episodes are rare before the age of 18 months, and only in rare instances where previous attacks can be identified is a recurrence after the age of 6 acceptable, and even then some doubt should be cast on the diagnosis. The differential diagnosis is of course the possibility of an epileptic tendency being unmasked by a fever, which carries a poorer long-term prognosis. True febrile convulsions rarely lead on to further forms of epilepsy. Therefore attention to detail in a suspected attack should be meticulous, as all long-term considerations depend on the accuracy of diagnosis.

The features that categorise febrile convulsions are:

(a) The onset of the attack should be the first indication that the child is unwell (i.e. the temperature rise has been extremely rapid). Fits occurring later in the day after a fever has started should be viewed with great suspicion.
(b) Only one attack per febrile episode should occur; further attacks on subsequent days are very suspect.
(c) No events should occur at any time *without a fever*, either prior to or subsequent to the suspected attack. The identification of

similar non-febrile episodes negates the diagnosis.

It follows from these considerations that no immediate treatment is necessary unless the convulsion is prolonged, as subsequent events are unlikely to occur during the same fever. There is no point in initiating antipyretic or anticonvulsant drugs during a fever because by the time a fever is identified the risk is already past. The major problem in a first attack is being certain that the cause of the fever is not meningitis or a cerebral abscess. Prompt identification of otitis media, tonsillitis, or an exanthem as an explanation for the fever is vital. If no cause is apparent, the possibility of primary neurological disease requires urgent exclusion with hospital referral.

Following recovery, there is considerable controversy as to whether prophylactic anticonvulsants are required and if so which is the preferred agent. It is the writer's view that no therapy is needed. Most affected children will only have three to four attacks over a 3- to 4-year period, and the disadvantages of 4 years' continuous anticonvulsant therapy have to be weighed against the low risk of repetition. Traditionally, phenobarbitone has been used, and claims for all major anticonvulsants have been made but with such low recurrence rates that it is difficult to get statistically valid evidence of the value of such treatment. A positive family history of the same disorder in older siblings or a parent adds to diagnostic certainty, and in such instances parents with knowledge of the disorder are usually unwilling to consider prophylactic medication.

The EEG is usually normal between attacks and the discovery of clear-cut epileptic abnormalities should cast some doubt on the diagnosis. A second attack should be awaited before initiating therapy, the situation being handled exactly as in idiopathic epilepsy. Most difficulties are experienced where sloppy criteria have failed to identify fits provoked by fever as the first evidence of an epileptic tendency. Studies claiming that febrile seizures are a common cause of brain damage often fail to identify clearly the possibility that the fever was an unmasking rather than a causal factor. This dilemma is unlikely to be resolved by further studies, and only by applying strict diagnostic criteria can patients who have a poor prognosis be identified, and regarded and treated from the outset as suffering from epilepsy.

## Recommendations for management

(a) A comprehensive personal and family history should be taken.

(b) No hospital referral is necessary unless the cause of the fever is uncertain or where there is evidence or suspicion of CNS infection.

(c) No specific therapy is needed unless the convulsion fails to subside, in which case intravenous diazepam (0.2 mg/kg) as a bolus injection is the treatment of choice. If intravenous injection is impossible, rectal diazepam (0.5 mg/kg) can be used. Because febrile convulsions are the commonest cause of status epilepticus in childhood, if the attack is not subsiding rapidly, diazepam should be given and urgent transfer to hospital arranged. In the vast majority of instances the seizure will have stopped before the doctor arrives, and no specific treatment is needed.

(d) If there is any doubt about the diagnosis, an EEG should be performed, and outpatient referral to the paediatric or neurological clinic is advisable.

(e) Any subsequent clinical events should be evaluated critically with the same care to exclude the possibility of epilepsy unmasked by a fever. The more frequent the attacks, the greater should be the suspicion that they are not simple febrile convulsions.

## PETIT MAL EPILEPSY (GENERALISED EPILEPSY WITHOUT CONVULSIONS)

Petit mal epilepsy is now classified as a generalised epilepsy without convulsion although variants containing some jerking movements, akinetic falls and automatisms are now included in this classification, which in the writer's view blurs the distinction between such attacks and complex partial seizures (temporal lobe or psychomotor seizures). In its classical form, petit mal consists of a brief, 5- to 15-seconds arrest of awareness, during which the *child* will stare and perhaps blink and the eyes may roll up, but he or she will then instantly recover and carry on as if nothing had happened, quite *unaware* of the event. This is a rare form of epilepsy (less than 2.5% of all epilepsy) which never starts *de novo* in adulthood. It is frequently misdiagnosed, and referral letters saying 'Please see this man of 54 who has developed petit mal', are both frequent and inevitably wrong!

The peak age of onset is between 4 and 10 years of age, although occasional examples are recognised before 12 months of age and some genuine examples may first be identified in the early teens. They are most frequently incorrectly identified in young patients who have short-lived complex partial seizures. The critical importance of this distinction used to lie in the therapy, some anti-petit mal drugs actually provoking grand mal attacks (trimethadione and ethosuximide) and some major anticonvulsants making petit mal worse and even capable of provoking petit mal status (sodium phenytoin and phenobarbitone). The current use of sodium valproate as the standard drug for petit mal has lessened this risk, as it provides protection against coincidental grand mal and seems not to provoke it. The prognosis of petit mal, if not complicated by other seizure types, is excellent, with 90% of sufferers attack-free by the late teens. Continuation of the attacks into adulthood is extremely unusual.

The EEG in petit mal is diagnostic. The main difficulty in interpretation lies in the fact that in *all* forms of epilepsy the standard epileptic discharge consists of a 2 to 3 cycles per second spike wave discharge, and if reported in this way is always assumed by non-experts to indicate petit mal. The value of the EEG in petit mal lies in the fact that not only are such discharges *always* found but they are *always* accompanied by a clinically observed attack, which should be noted on the record by the technician. If no external evidence of an episode is witnessed, the technician will write 'nil seen' on the record. This latter comment excludes petit mal. A great many of the diagnostic errors mentioned in this section are the result of an inaccurate history, compounded by ignorance of this essential feature of the EEG. It should always be possible to report 'the EEG is diagnostic of petit mal'.

### The major problems of petit mal

(a) Failure to identify petit mal, where attacks can occur 60 times an hour, may lead to serious learning problems.
(b) Inappropriate medication may make attacks worse or provoke major convulsions.
(c) Incorrect identification (i.e. the attacks are actually complex partial seizures) dramatically alters the prognosis. Such children, far from becoming free of attacks by their early teens, go on to develop more typical complex partial seizures and

grand mal attacks in puberty. Adult neurologists are particularly sensitive to the wrath of parents in this situation, who have been presented with the favourable prognosis of petit mal only to find the unwanted reappearance of a more serious form of epilepsy in the child's early teens.

Because of these problems it is difficult to be certain of the exact risk of children with pure, correctly diagnosed petit mal developing other forms of epilepsy. The initial diagnosis seems to have been incorrect so often in those cases where other attacks appear that petit mal occurring in association with other seizure types in the same child is probably a very rare event and should only be accepted after very critical review of the whole case.

The treatment of choice for petit mal has become sodium valproate in a dose of 200–500 mg tds. Ethosuximide 250–500 mg tds may have a place in resistant cases, but the risk of provoking other seizure types may require simultaneous therapy with sodium valproate to minimise this risk. Once the child has had no observed attacks for 2 years, treatment can be withdrawn and the child should be observed. Unnecessary continuation of ethosuximide into adulthood is an occasional cause of continuing major epilepsy (see below).

Petit mal status epilepticus presents as an ongoing bemused befuddled state with drooling, little jolts of the head and fluttering of the eyes and eyelids. It is a rare condition. It may occasionally be the presenting symptom of petit mal and may cause considerable diagnostic confusion until an EEG has been performed. It is not a life-threatening condition and can continue for several days until diagnosed and treated without the child coming to harm. It may respond to rebreathing from a paper bag, and if this fails intravenous (0.2 mg/kg) or rectal (0.5 mg/kg) diazepam should be effective or as an alternative lorazepam (0.05–0.2 mg/kg). Both diazepam and lorazepam should be infused at a rate not exceeding 2 mg/min, and respiration must be carefully monitored.

## COMPLEX PARTIAL SEIZURES (FORMERLY TEMPORAL LOBE EPILEPSY, PSYCHOMOTOR EPILEPSY)

These episodes are now classified under several rubrics of the focal epilepsy group, categorised by the nature of the aura involved, including the full range of motor, sensory, intellectual, gustatory, olfactory, auditory, visual or almost any other functional disorder occurring as part of an attack of altered or lost awareness, which may remain circumscribed or progress to a generalised convulsion. Perhaps those most readily suspected are episodes preceded by altered taste or smell, and the extreme brevity of such phenomena should be stressed. Similarly a feeling of coldness in the perineum or a rising feeling in the epigastrium are quite common visceral phenomena. In all instances, the suddenness of onset, followed by alteration of awareness and observed automatic movements such as chewing, munching, lip-smacking, fiddling with clothing and walking aimlessly, followed by a period of confusion and uncertainty on recovery, characterise the attack. In the recovery stage, some irritability and aggressive tendencies may be demonstrated but the extreme rarity of complex co-ordinated aggressive action is important to note.

Complex partial seizures constitute the most common form of epilepsy, and in view of their diversity can sometimes elude diagnosis for years. In some instances the peculiarity of the attack may inhibit the patient from seeking advice. These attacks can occur at any age and in childhood are readily confused with petit mal. In the adult, patients seen following their first major convulsion will often, on close questioning, give a history of events of this sort occurring over many years, the significance of which had hitherto escaped attention. Often the cessation of such attacks following effective treatment directed at prevention of further major episodes identifies their nature and confirms the effectiveness of treatment.

Such attacks are typically random. In females an association with period times is frequently cited. In both sexes, a relationship to stress and mealtimes is often noted and inexplicable. If major attacks occur, they may follow such a complex partial event or occur without warning. In all age groups the frequent eventual appearance of major attacks is important to note. It is often an attack that first prompts referral in many instances. A child with this condition, incorrectly identified as suffering from petit mal, will often have its first major episode at puberty. Adults after many years of such episodes, during which time they have driven and worked without incident and injury, suddenly find their driving and livelihood jeopardised by the identification of these attacks following their first major seizure. Prognostically complex partial seizures are the type of attack least likely to subside spontaneously and are the most resistant to complete control with medication.

The EEG in temporal lobe epilepsy can be extremely difficult.

Typical spike wave discharges, often starting asymmetrically but rapidly spreading to both sides, would constitute a fairly straightforward confirmatory finding. As noted earlier, this can easily be misinterpreted as indicating petit mal. Focal spikes in one or other temporal lead probably provide the most unequivocal confirmation of the diagnosis and location of the abnormal discharges. In many instances the EEG on a standard recording will be normal. The yield of abnormal findings may be increased by a sleep recording or the use of sphenoidal or oesophageal leads. The recent advent of telemetered and continuous recording EEG has increased the likelihood of picking up infrequent discharges in such patients.

Treatment is difficult. Of the older agents primidone (Mysoline) is probably the most successful agent and may still have a place in intractable cases. The main drawback is poor tolerance, producing drowsiness and ataxia in a surprisingly high proportion of patients. The dose range is 125–500 mg tds starting with very low doses (125 mg nocte) and gradually increasing to tolerance. It should not be used in patients allergic to barbiturates, and may cause behavioural disturbance in children. Phenytoin (Epanutin) can be a successful treatment but in rare cases may actually provoke complex partial seizures and this possibility should always be considered if no response is seen or if attacks appear to worsen. Ethosuximide has no place in the management of this type of attack and may indeed provoke episodes. Any adult patient still taking this drug may well be continuing to have attacks because of this provocative effect, and withdrawal is recommended.

Several drugs have been introduced for the treatment of complex partial seizures and subsequently withdrawn, but two more recent agents have established an important place in therapy.

Carbamazepine (Tegretol) is probably the most successful and has become the drug of choice when initiating treatment. A wide dose range of 100–400 mg tds gives considerable flexibility, and even intractable cases may respond to very small doses if this agent has not previously been tried. The drug is well tolerated. Marrow depression is rare but cutaneous reactions are not uncommon and may be severe. Patients should be advised to stop the drug immediately if skin irritation occurs.

Sodium valproate is the second drug of choice with a wide dose range of 200–1000 mg tds, giving dose flexibility. Clinical control does not correlate well with blood levels, and problems such as hair loss, tremor, weight gain, indigestion and potentially fatal liver damage all require careful consideration.

Less certain agents of occasional value are the benzodiazepine derivatives clonazepam (Rivotril) and clobazam (Frisium). Both have the potential disadvantage of sedation and may enhance the sedative effect of other agents. Clonazepam is used in a dose of 0.25–2 mg tds. It should be introduced in low dosage and increased if lack of sedation permits. If no effect is apparent, it should be withdrawn as there is no useful interaction with other agents to justify its continuation. Clobazam is used in a dose of 10 mg at night or 10 mg bd; daytime sedation is the disadvantage of the latter. As a supplement to carbamazepine it may enable complete control to be established. It is claimed that the benefit wanes over several months but this has not been a problem in the writer's experience and this drug combined with carbamazepine would be my current treatment of choice for this type of epilepsy.

The difficulty of obtaining complete control and the advent of major attacks in patients suffering from complex partial seizures often leads to polypharmacy. There is a natural reluctance to discontinue a partially effective drug while introducing another, and a patient may finally be taking three or four agents simultaneously with complete drug interactions and side effects and sometimes surprisingly little benefits. However, complete control of such attacks with a single agent is extremely hard to achieve, and the modern trend to monotherapy must not be allowed to dominate thinking so much that the use of more than one agent is not attempted.


## COMPLEX PARTIAL SEIZURE STATUS EPILEPTICUS

This situation is fairly rare. It may produce a stuporose drooling state as in petit mal, or a prolonged, near psychotic state with zombie-like behaviour, including complex automatisms, and a psychiatric condition may be suspected. Treatment with intravenous diazepam is usually effective but may have to be repeated on several occasions before the episode abates (diazepam 5–10 mg IVI, repeated in 30 minutes). Intravenous phenytoin may also be used if the patient is not already taking this drug.

## GRAND MAL EPILEPSY (GENERALISED CONVULSIVE EPILEPSY)

Grand mal epilepsy is characterised by loss of consciousness and falling, usually accompanied by convulsive movements of tonic then clonic type and occasionally complicated by incontinence of urine or faeces.

It is a form of epilepsy that may occur at any age and is certainly the type most readily identified. Unfortunately it is occasionally *too* easily identified when a patient who merely stiffens during a syncopal attack is incorrectly diagnosed as suffering from grand mal epilepsy. Grand mal epilepsy carries considerable potential risk of injury but in general it is surprising how rarely serious injury occurs.

There is usually no premonitory warning other than in those cases where a complex partial seizure culminates in a grand mal attack. Although attacks could theoretically occur quite randomly, a very high proportion are nocturnal, frequently in the hour before awakening and less commonly just after going to sleep. The advent of attacks later in the day without specific provocation such as an afternoon nap bodes badly for the chances of control. Such attacks carry increased hazard and introduce the problems of sedation because of the high doses of medication required during working hours. A careful history should always document the diurnal and nocturnal pattern of attacks. The tendency for attacks to remain purely nocturnal is recognised in the driving regulations that permit patients to continue to drive despite having epileptic attacks provided that such attacks remain purely nocturnal for over three years. Focal features occurring at the onset of, during or subsequent to the attack should be carefully noted as such features greatly increase the risk of underlying pathology.

Provocative factors should be sought and include excess alcohol, exceptionally late nights, sleep deprivation due to travel or illness and potentially epileptogenic medication such as antihistamines, antidepressants and major tranquillisers. The clear identification of a provocative factor unlikely to be repeated may allow the first episode to be regarded as a 'one off' attack. In purely nocturnal cases, suspicion alone may justify the diagnosis. Evidence, such as a wet bed, bitten tongue, black eye or falls from the bed, can often be identified in retrospect. This often follows the first documentation of nocturnal epilepsy, when the patient shares a bedroom with a relative or friend.

In every case, the events of the 24 hours prior to the attack, and the time, location, nature and duration of the episode are all essential to accurate diagnosis. One of the most frequent dilemmas is the syncopal attack that culminates in a witnessed seizure. This is often compounded by the tendency for such attacks to occur in dental surgeries, during immunisation procedures or while visiting relatives in hospital and therefore to be witnessed by paramedical staff, whose diagnosis of epilepsy is too readily accepted as correct and difficult to dismiss. Very few doctors have actually witnessed enough epileptic events to be as dogmatic as the retired district nurse, whose dogmatism is equalled only by her lack of experience of such events.

The hallmark of this particular situation is the provoking event and the circumstances. Trauma, such as a kicked shin, a cut finger, a chisel through the hand, the sight of blood or lying on a dentist's couch, may all provoke precipitate fainting. A ghoulish or medical film. first-aid demonstration or someone else vomiting can all provoke syncope in observers. Hot, stuffy rooms, restaurants, cinemas and theatres, parties and job interviews are common locations, especially if additional factors such as dysmenorrhoea or psychological stress are operative.

A classical syndrome with visual blurring, muffled hearing, goose pimples, feeling very hot and sweaty but becoming very pale and clammy, will make diagnosis easy. Sometimes, and this is where circumstantial evidence is crucial, the patient will collapse without warning. Under such circumstances, generalised stiffening and fine trembling, as if shivering with cold, are the rule and these features are aggravated if the patient is allowed to remain upright. This is the situation so often misdiagnosed as a convulsion. Such is the impact of an epileptic fit on a person's life, driving and employment that an incorrect diagnosis may be completely life-wrecking and the balance of doubt should always be exercised in the patient's favour.

This subject has been covered in such detail because it is such a common problem and diagnostic mistakes are so frequent and devastating for the patient.

A grand mal epilepic fit should be quite unmistakable, as a set sequence of events is the rule. The warning, if any, is so brief that the patient rarely has time to attempt to sit or lie down, and indeed any comment from the patient that they are about to collapse should immediately cast doubt on the diagnosis. Consciousness is suddenly and completely lost, and if unsupported the patient may fall. If sitting in a chair they may merely slump and for a few seconds will appear to have gone to sleep. The patient will then develop a tonic spasm, sometimes severe enough for an involuntary cry to be emitted. The eyes will stare and roll up into the head, and the head may extend or rotate to one or other side. The arms will usually stiffen to the sides with the fists clenched and the legs extended. The duration of this phase is usually some 30 to 40 seconds, during which the face will flush and then become cyanotic. If the tongue is between the teeth, it will be bitten, incontinence of urine or faeces may occur, and in occasional cases crush fractures of vertebrae may result from the force of the spasm. Suddenly the patient will go limp. After a brief pause, of perhaps 15 to 30 seconds, rhythmic jerking in all four limbs will begin and the head may jerk backwards. This results in the back of the head and the heels banging on the ground in unison. This phase may continue for 2 to 3 minutes but is the part of the attack that may be prolonged or become continuous in status epilepticus (see below). On recovery the patient is invariably confused and drowsy and may go straight into a deep sleep. If strenuous attempts are made to awaken them, they may react aggressively.

The most important differential diagnosis is the possibility of a simulated attack or 'pseudo-seizure'. This is a surprisingly common problem, and a high proportion of patients with apparently intractable or uncontrollable epilepsy are found to have this condition on careful reinvestigation. The main clue to this diagnosis lies in the nature of the attack, but when someone is apparently convulsing in a particularly dramatic way, panic reigns and the possibility of non-organicity is rarely considered.

The typical features of a 'pseudo-seizure' are as follows:

(a) The attacks are entirely random and usually occur in public, where they will make maximum impact. In the last 15 years in my clinics, the only seizures occurring in the waiting room have been of this type!

(b) The patient will often scream and shout in a more organised way than the brief cry of epilepsy.

(c) In the tonic phase, back arching into an opisthotonic position is so common as to be diagnostic. In the clonic phase, the movements are desynchronised and may assume aggressive qualities, deliberately kicking or punching bystanders. The head typically flails from side to side, not up and down. The eyes are clenched tightly shut and are resistant to passive opening. The plantar responses are flexor but the examiner will be fortunate not to be kicked in the process.

(d) It is not unusual for patients to quote back comments made about them *during* the fit.

Perhaps one of the most difficult situations in this whole field is when a patient with genuine epilepsy starts to simulate attacks for gain or effect, or where someone with a close knowledge of epilepsy, with an affected relative or friend, produces mimicked episodes. An EEG immediately after or during the attack is normal, and a serum prolactin level should be within normal limits. The serum prolactin level rises appreciably after a genuine convulsion, and a blood specimen taken by the general practitioner at the scene of a suspected event may provide invaluable help in confirming or casting doubt on the nature of the attack.

Interpretation of the EEG in grand mal epilepsy is especially difficult. There are three main possibilities:

(a) It may be entirely normal. This is often the case after a nocturnal event, and can lead to the diagnosis being disputed or may lead to unjustified reassurance.
(b) It may be grossly abnormal and show clear-cut evidence of a long-standing epileptic tendency with frequent epileptic bursts of spike-wave type. This provides indisputable confirmation of the diagnosis.
(c) It may show a focal abnormality often in one or other temporal region, which may not only provide support for the diagnosis of epilepsy, but may raise the suspicion of an underlying causal lesion and prompt immediate further investigation.

Although at first sight a normal EEG may appear reassuring, it is very wise to do repeat studies at 6 month intervals. The writer has had several patients in this category, who have harboured tumours with initially normal EEGs. The grossly abnormal epileptic EEG is the most reassuring. It is not associated with underlying structural disease, and surprisingly often such patients' attacks are the most easily controlled. There is no need to repeatedly confirm that the EEG in these cases remains abnormal, and it is a popular misconception that successful treatment is accompanied by an improved EEG and that repeated EEGs can indicate how the patient is progressing. Only the occurrence of further fits can indicate this.

The treatment of grand mal epilepsy is perhaps the most flexible in the whole field. It is important to realise that all anticonvulsants can provoke fits at toxic levels. Occasional patients are encountered where, even in therapeutic range, an anticonvulsant can provoke rather than prevent their episodes. If a patient is convinced that his or her attacks are worse in spite of treatment, this possibility must be urgently considered.

Phenytoin is the single most used agent, in a dose of 200–400 mg daily. One of its major advantages is the slow metabolism and long half-life which give a built-in safety margin in the event of a missed dose. Although potential side effects are numerous, with the exception of cutaneous hypersensitivity it is extremely unusual to have to discontinue the drug. It is important to be aware of the acute glandular fever or lymphoma-like syndrome that can occur in some patients taking phenytoin. Serious diagnostic confusion may occur in such instances. In many trials sodium valproate has demonstrated similar effectiveness in controlling grand mal when used as a single agent (dosage 200–500 mg tds). Carbamazepine has also shown equal potency (dosage 100–400 mg tds). Primidone is an effective agent but poorly tolerated by a sufficiently high proportion of patients to limit its use as a first-line drug.

The treatment of choice is a single agent of personal preference used in a dose adequate to prevent further attacks and monitored by blood levels if control is not immediately apparent. It should be stressed that getting the agent into the so-called therapeutic range is not necessarily accompanied by successful control and in some instances complete control is apparent before the blood level reaches this range. In these instances, commonsense should prevail, as the object is to prevent fits and not necessarily produce a specific level in the blood. If attacks are purely nocturnal, a single large dose on retiring may be sufficient. It is traditional to use a smaller dose of the same agent in the day as a 'top up' but this is not strictly necessary unless daytime attacks emerge. It should be stressed that there is very little indication for the use of phenobarbitone, which has unacceptable side effects on concentration, memory and behaviour compared with modern agents. Its use as a spansule containing 60 or 100 mg at night may have a limited place in nocturnal epilepsy occurring on wakening, when a single agent has proved ineffective. If phenobarbitone has been used in a regime, withdrawal may be very difficult. Not only may psychological withdrawal symptoms such as tremor and insomnia occur, but, in addition, withdrawal fits are very common. Such fits are often assumed by the patient and sometimes their doctors as confirming the miraculous efficacy of this drug rather than recognising its shortcomings and the dangers of sudden discontinuation. Withdrawal should be covered by the use of a sedative agent such as clobazam 10 mg nocte.

## GRAND MAL STATUS EPILEPTICUS

This is the most serious complication of epilepsy and still carries a mortality rate of 10%. It exists when an attack is continuous for over 30 minutes or consciousness is not regained between a series of individual major convulsions. The immediate risk is of airway obstruction due to inhalation of blood or vomit leading to cerebral anoxia or subsequent chest infection. If seizures continue, cerebral oedema, hypoglycaemia, and exhaustion may ensue.

The cause may remain obscure, and if a patient not known to be epileptic presents as status epilepticus, the risk of an underlying frontal neoplasm is sufficiently high (about 50%) to prompt immediate further investigation. Missed medication, intercurrent illness, severe vomiting or diarrhoea or the inadvertent prescription of potentially epileptogenic agents or alcohol abuse can be the cause. Rarely, new intracranial pathology, such as meningitis, cerebral tumour or cerebrovascular accident (CVA) may be responsible.

(a) The usual immediate management of the unconscious patient should be initiated, with airway control the priority, by oropharyngeal airway or by intubation if necessary. An intravenous line should be established. Preliminary investigation should include careful history from friends and relatives, examination for evidence of the possible cause, and appropriate blood tests, including anticonvulsant levels.

(b) A dextrose infusion with added vitamin B1 if alcoholism is suspected should be given via the intravenous line.

(c) Diazepam, 10 mg by intravenous injection at a rate of 2 mg per minute should be given and may be repeated once within 15 minutes if seizures recur. Respiration should be carefully monitored during this phase. A maximum dose of 20 mg only should be given during the first hour. In the adult, lorazepam 4–8 mg at a rate of 2 mg/min via the infusion line or clonazepam in a dose of 1 mg given over 30 seconds are suitable alternatives. Although perhaps slower in onset of action than diazepam, it is thought that a longer duration of action may have a significant advantage in preventing subsequent relapse.

(d) Subsequent measures vary considerably in different units and different countries. In Great Britain, parenteral phenytoin and both short- and long-acting barbiturates are not popular, although they seem to be frequently used as second-line agents in the USA. Paraldehyde 10 ml, given as 5 ml in the upper outer quadrant of each buttock, is possibly the best treatment if diazepam fails. The paraldehyde must be fresh from an unopened ampoule. Badly stored paraldehyde can depolymerise to acetaldehyde and oxidise to acetic acid, and 7 ml of such a solution can be fatal. It must be given by glass syringe, carefully injected to avoid sciatic nerve damage, and may be repeated as 5 ml 4-hourly over the next 12 hours. It is highly effective, if somewhat unpleasant in use.

(e) Chlormethiazole, by intravenous infusion, is a suitable alternative, but has the disadvantage of being highly irritant and has to be administered via a central venous line. It is supplied as a 0.8% solution and is used at a drop rate of 10–60 drops per minute. Treatment is started at 60 drops per minute (4 ml/32 mg) and the drip rate is adjusted down to ten drops per minute determined by the control of attacks. This may have to be continued for several days.

(f) Lignocaine 1–2 mg/kg per hour may be given by intravenous infusion in a 0.2% solution. This may cause respiratory depression but, even more worrying, can actually provoke status epilepticus. It is therefore difficult on the present evidence to recommend this as a standard treatment.

(g) For fear of toxicity parenteral phenytoin cannot be used in patients already on the drug and the recommended stat dose of 120 mg intravenously, given at a rate of 50 mg per minute, has caused irreversible cerebellar toxicity. The difficulty with the use of barbiturates is that general anaesthetic doses are required, and when the agent is allowed to wear off, withdrawal seizures may well cause the patient to revert to status epilepticus.

(h) Where fits are poorly controlled and the patient is becoming anoxic for lengthy periods, neuromuscular blockade, with positive pressure ventilation, may be necessary. This has the disadvantage of concealing the fits and making further clinical evaluation impossible. In the last 15 years, the writer has not had to look for measures beyond diazepam, paraldehyde or chlormethiazole in any patient in status epilepticus.

Accurate diagnosis, correct EEG interpretation and the use of appropriate anticonvulsants in effective dosage are the basis of good epileptic management. The condition can destroy the morale and career of the sufferer and can on rare occasions threaten life. Control of epilepsy is one of the most dramatic and satisfying accomplishments in medicine.

## FURTHER READING

Bleck, T.P. and Klawans, H.L. (1986) Neurologic emergencies. *Med. Clin. N. Amer.* *70*, 1168–83

Delgado-Escueta, A.V. and Treiman, D.M. (1985) The emergency treatment of status epilepticus. In R.T. Johnson (ed.),*Current therapy in neurologic disease*, C. V. Mosby, St. Louis, Mo., pp. 51–61

Pedley, T.A. and Meldrum, B.S. (eds) (1983) *Recent advances in epilepsy 1*, Churchill Livingstone, Edinburgh

Pedley, T.A. and Meldrum, B.S. (eds) (1985) *Recent advances in epilepsy 2*. Churchill Livingstone, Edinburgh

Porter, R.J. and Morselli, P.L. (eds) (1985) *The epilepsies*, Butterworth, London

Rawal, K. and D'Souza, B.J. (1985) Status epilepticus. *Critical Care Clinics 1*, 339–53

Tyrer, J.H. (ed.) (1980) *The treatment of epilepsy: current status of modern therapy*, Vol. 5, MTP Press, Lancaster

# 7

# Infection of the Nervous System

Bruce Moffatt and Daniel F. Hanley

## BACTERIAL MENINGITIS

The diagnosis and treatment of bacterial infection of the cerebrospinal fluid space represents a neurological emergency. Successful treatment rests on early detection and rapid initiation of appropriate therapy. The usual clinical presentation of meningitis is fever, headache, meningismus and neurological dysfunction. The neurological signs may be focal or diffuse. Usually they are diffuse and mild, such as indifference, lethargy, or confusion. In infants these altered mental states are likely to present as lack of interest in feeding and excessive somnolence. Frequently the patient will rapidly progress to delirium, coma and/or seizures (either focal or generalised).

Historical evidence of sinus or otitic infection or neurosurgical procedure is important information to obtain as it may alter the initial antibiotic regimen. This information is best obtained from a family member and should be investigated further during the physical examination. Patients presenting with a meningitis symptom complex should have a complete but rapid physical evaluation for thoracic, abdominal, soft tissue and parameningeal sources of infection followed by a thorough and rapid neurological evaluation. Special attention should be paid to possible focal neurological findings. When there is no obvious aetiology for fever and no evidence of a focal cerebral lesion, the patient should have an immediate lumbar puncture. For patients with focal findings or evidence of possible intracranial hypertension such as papilloedema, computed tomography should be performed on an emergent basis. When computed tomography is not available and the patient presents with frank neurological dysfunction and meningismus, initiation of antibiotic therapy and transport to the nearest centre for appropriate critical (intensive) care should be arranged.

Cerebrospinal fluid should be obtained for gram stain, culture, antibiotic sensitivity, antigen identification, cell count, protein and glucose. An aliquot of CSF should be examined microscopically, after centrifugation and gram stain, by the physician responsible for the patient. Patients with either a CSF polymorphonuclear leucocytosis or any neurological abnormalities (particularly alterations of consciousness) and equivocal CSF findings should be started on antibiotic therapy appropriate for probable meningitis. The initial choice of antibiotic is best based on the age of the patient, the presence or absence of associated infections, and the epidemiology of local microorganism drug resistance. The most common clinical grouping of patients is newborns (< 2 months), young children (2 months–5 years) and older patients (> 5 years). Gram-negative meningitis is particularly common in the newborn group, with *E. coli*, *Proteus*, *Haemophilus*, beta streptococci and *Listeria monocytogenes* being common organisms. These microorganisms are apparently acquired at the time of birth from the female genital tract. Young children have a high incidence of *Haemophilus influenzae* meningitis. *Streptococcus pneumonia* and *Neisseria meningitides* also occur in this age group. The incidence of bacterial meningitis is lower at all other ages, and *Streptococcus pneumoniae* and *Neisseria meningitides* are the most common organisms. Gram-negative bacterial meningitis can occur in the paediatric age group > 2 months, particularly in hospitalised patients, but is more common in adults over the age of 60 years. For both age groups the common community-acquired organisms include *E. coli*, *Haemophilus*, *Proteus* and *Klebsiella*. For the hospitalised patient *Enterobacter*, *Pseudomonas aeruginosa*, other *Acinetobacter* species and *Serratia* infections are also commonly identified and are often resistant to the usual levels of antibiotics. Patients who develop meningitis following a neurosurgical procedure are likely to be infected with an organism acquired at the time of the procedure. These include *Staphylococcus epidermidis*, *S. loccocus aureus*, oropharyngeal organisms (streptococci, pneumococci and *Haemophilus*) and less commonly gram-negative organisms such as *E. coli*, *Klebsiella*, *Pseudomonas* and *Proteus*.

Timely initiation of antibiotic therapy and the appropriate range of microorganism coverage are important factors in producing an optimal outcome. The physician identifying a patient with probable meningitis should be responsible for initiating intravenous antibiotic therapy. It may be necessary to consult other experienced physicians regarding the best combination of antibiotics, but this should be done without delay in the initiation of therapy.

Neonates should receive ampicillin and an aminoglycoside as most gram-negative rods are susceptible to this combination, as are *Listeria* and streptococci. For children, particularly those of 5 years and younger where *Haemophilus* influenza is the most likely community acquired infection, ampicillin and chloramphenicol provide the best initial opportunity to treat drug-resistant stains. When the infection is acquired in the hospital, gram-negative organisms should also be treated with an aminoglycoside or cephalosporin in combination with ampicillin. This regimen is probably equally appropriate for adult patients with either community- or hospital-acquired meningitis. Consideration of the possibility of drug-resistant nosocomial gram-negative meningitis may require the addition of newer beta-lactamase-resistant penicillin or cephalosporin. Choosing an additional drug in this situation is often uniquely dependent on the drug-susceptibility pattern of the expected hospital-acquired nosocomial infection. When the child or adult in question has undergone a neurosurgical procedure in the last 4 to 8 weeks, a penicillinase-resistant drug with activity against *Staphylococcus* such as nafcillin or vancomycin should be started in combination with an aminoglycoside and a drug specific for likely nosocomial gram-negative meningitis (Table 7.1).

General medical support should be started urgently. For the severely ill patient, airway and circulatory compromise are likely. Arterial pressure and intracranial pressure monitoring may be helpful in complicated cases. Seizures should be treated prophylactically with phenytoin 18 mg/kg IV. Studies to define the presence of a coagulopathy should also be performed. Subsequent care should be directed at maintaining adequate antibiotic levels. This is best assessed with minimum bacteriocidal concentration studies against the causative organism. Repeat lumbar puncture is best performed 24 to 48 hours after initiation of therapy. At this time a sterile culture is often attained for gram-positive meningitis. The presence of a drug-resistant organism and the levels of cerebrospinal fluid antibiotics can be assessed at this time. A favourable clinical course including resolution of fever, improved mentation, cardiopulmonary stability and the absence of focal neurological signs are probably the best indicators of therapeutic efficacy. For patients who respond clinically, 10 to 14 days of antibiotics is usually adequate. The laboratory demonstration of microorganism sensitivity to the levels

**Table 7.1**: Treatment of meningitis

| | Initial regimen | For a complicated clinical course consider: |
|---|---|---|
| Neonate | Ampicillin 200–300 mg/kg/day<br>Gentamicin 10–15 mg/kg/day | Cefotaxime 200–300 mg/kg/day |
| Child | Ampicillin 150–400 mg/kg/day<br>Chloramphenicol 100 mg/kg/day | Cefotaxime 200–300 mg/kg/day |
| Adult (community-acquired) | Ampicillin 12–16 g/day plus<br>Gentamicin 5 mg/kg/day or<br>Cefotaxime 12 g/day | Amikacin 15 mg/kg/day |
| Adult (hospital-acquired) | Ampicillin 12–16 g/day<br>Amikacin 15 mg/kg/day plus<br>Cefotaxime 12 g/day | Pipericillin 30 g/day |
| Child or adult (hospital-acquired post head trauma or neurosurgery) | Nafcillin 12–16 g/day<br>Amikacin 15 mg/kg/day<br>Cefotaxime 150–200 mg/kg/day | Vancomycin 2 g/day and/or<br>Pipericillin 30 g/day |

of drug employed provides helpful confirmation of such a clinical response. Brain abscess and/or subdural empyema represent the most common sites of poorly resolved infection. Computed tomography is a sensitive test to define these complications and can be used as a guide to define the length of prolonged therapy. The presence of sinusitis or osteomyelitis will also dictate a longer treatment course, often 4 to 8 weeks. Adequate drainage of all focal sources of infection and removal of contaminated foreign bodies should be performed when these complications are identified.

Meningitis is frequently associated with fatality. For both neonates and adults over 45 years, US national case fatality ratios are 20% or more depending on the organism. For children and adults from 1 month to 45 years the mortality is about 10%. More detailed clinical prediction of the likely outcome is not presently possible. Early diagnosis and treatment remain the cornerstone of medical intervention.

## BASILAR SKULL FRACTURE

Recognised basilar skull fracture accompanies about 25% of all head trauma that comes to medical attention. It usually follows blunt head trauma that is associated with loss of consciousness, but may follow seemingly insignificant head injury. Basilar skull fracture can be recognised by the presence of periorbital ecchymosis, Battle's sign, haemotympanum, or anosmia. Its importance as an infectious risk is associated with the potential for a dural fistula and associated cerebrospinal fluid (CSF) leak. About 10% of basilar skull fractures are associated with a CSF leak, and between 2 and 9% are complicated by the development of meningitis.

The CSF leak begins in the majority of cases within 48 hours of head trauma and is announced by the presence of otorrhoea or rhinorrhoea. However, the first sign of a dural fistula may not be a demonstrable CSF leak but may begin with meningitis itself. The occurrence of otorrhoea or rhinorrhoea may be delayed if a blood clot or swollen brain occludes the fistula. Occasionally the leak may start weeks or months following the trauma, so that eliciting a history of any type of head trauma is important in a patient presenting with an otherwise 'spontaneous' CSF leak.

The diagnosis of otorrhoea is straightforward after a careful examination of the tympanic membrane has been made. Rhinorrhoea can be obvious, but is often difficult to diagnose. The CSF protein is low and therefore presents as a more watery fluid than the viscous nasal secretion. If nasal discharge is found, collecting some of it on filter paper may reward the examiner with a 'double ring' sign as the CSF forms an outer ring about a central circle of blood. Testing the fluid for glucose may be helpful as CSF has a higher glucose than nasal secretions (more than 30 mg/dl).

When positive, the clinical examination is usually all that is needed to make the diagnosis of a basilar skull fracture. However, because the signs and symptoms may be delayed in onset, other tests are often used. Plain X-ray is usually not helpful as even when the appropriate films are taken, only 30–40% basilar skull fractures are demonstrable. CT scanning is better, but it can be negative in the presence of a clinically obvious basilar skull fracture. Fluid in a sinus or the presence of intracranial air (pneumocephalus) are occasionally seen. Pneumocephalus on plain X-ray has been associated with a 50% risk of CSF leak and 25% risk of meningitis. Because the CT scan can detect much less intracranial air than plain X-ray, the presence of pneumocephalus is now more frequently noted. This finding reflects the presence of at least a transient dural fistula and an increased risk of meningitis.

The source of meningitis associated with basilar skull fracture is thought to come from the paranasal and mastoid sinuses which are often breeched by the basilar skull fracture. Approximately two-thirds of meningitis cases associated with basilar skull fracture are caused by *Streptococcus* (*S. pneumoniae* or other species); *Haemophilus influenzae* is the next most common. Enteric gram-negative bacilli are rarely the cause of meningitis in this setting. The onset of meningitis following the CSF leak is usually less than one month. Relapsing or recurrent meningitis is occasionally seen in the setting of the dural fistula.

The majority of CSF leaks close spontaneously within two weeks and require no special therapy. Conservative management of the CSF leaks include bed rest with elevation of the head, avoiding straining and coughing, stool softeners, acetazolamide to slow CSF production, and in more persistent leaks serial lumbar punctures or a temporary lumbar drain. A persistent leak should alert one to the potential presence of hydrocephalus. This often requires a permanent lumbar–peritoneal or ventricular–peritoneal shunt.

For basilar skull fractures the use of prophylactic antibiotics is controversial and the efficacy of prophylaxis remains unresolved. A prospective, randomised, double-blind study failed to demonstrate a benefit from their use. Furthermore, if prophylactic antibiotics are used, the selection of a drug-resistant organism may occur. Basilar skull fractures are not treated prophylactically at the authors' institution. However, if evidence of meningitis is significant, nafcillin (2 g IV q. 4 hours) and chloramphenicol (1 g IV q. 6 hours) are begun. This regimen is altered in accordance with culture results and antibiotic sensitivity.

Because basilar skull fractures are common after head trauma and because CSF leaks carry a significant risk of meningitis, it is prudent to observe all basilar skull fracture patients for CSF leaks for 48–72 hours. This is the period of major risk for the development of a CSF leak. If a leak is a noted, more prolonged close observation for signs of meningitis is mandatory.

Non-traumatic dural fistulae are uncommon, but are occasionally associated with chronic hydrocephalus, congenital anomalies (encephaloceles) or mass lesions (tumours and cysts). Patients presenting with such fistulae should receive an evaluation to determine the site and cause of the leak. This typically includes sinus X-ray, a head CT, metrizamide or isotope cisternography with

CT and an LP. Surgical therapy is often required to stop the leak.

## POST-OPERATIVE INFECTION

Even with the use of perioperative prophylactic antibiotics, post-operative infection complicates craniotomy in 0.3 to 0.5% of cases. It is usually caused by organisms introduced at the time of surgery, but may also arise from a perioperative bacteraemia. The leading organisms are *Staphylococcus aureus* and gram-negative bacilli. The signs and symptoms are similar to those found in acute bacterial meningitis, but the course may also be a more protracted one. It should be noted that most neurosurgical patients receive corticosteroids in doses that limit or delay inflammatory symptoms. Diagnosis depends on obtaining a CSF sample. For many neuro-surgical patients, a spinal tap is inadvisable due to elevated intracranial pressure (ICP) or mass effect. Ventricular fluid samples can be helpful in some of these situations. The results of the CSF sample should guide therapy. A gram stain is positive in the majority of infections. However, if the gram stain is negative in the setting of a clinical suspicion of infection and a CSF leucocytosis, broad-spectrum antibiotics should be initiated empirically. Counter-immunoelectrophoresis is frequently able to detect the presence of bacterial antigen in CSF . This technique provides information helpful to the proper selection of antibiotics.

## SHUNT INFECTIONS

Ventricular–peritoneal and ventricular–atrial shunt insertion predispose patients to a higher risk of CNS infection. These probably occur via contamination at the time of insertion and are usually evident within the first two months post-operatively. The majority of infections are caused by *Staphylococcus epidermidis* and diphtheroid bacteria; occasionally other normal skin flora are responsible. Since most infections are caused by low-grade pathogens, the resultant clinical course is usually subacute or chronic. As with any foreign body, the shunt may be seeded during bacteraemia and can harbour other organisms: *Staphylococcus aureus*, *Streptococcus pneumoniae*, *Haemophilus influenzae* or gram-negative rods. Both acute and chronic shunt infections are typically marked by a temperature elevation, malaise, failure to thrive, and/or signs or elevated intracranial pressure (headache, nausea and vomiting, bradycardia). Diagnosis is made by taping the shunt and is confirmed by repeat cultures. Initial treatment with nafcillin or vancomycin is frequent. Additional antibiotics should be directed by the gram stain and culture results. Cure is based on sterilising the CSF, removal of the infected shunt and subsequent replacement.

## EPIDURAL/SUBDURAL INFECTIONS

### Cranial sites

Epidural abscess and subdural empyema represent rare infections of potential intracranial spaces. The epidural abscess is an infection arising between the calvarium and dura. The subdural empyema refers to an infection in the space between the dura and arachnoid. The epidural abscess causes signs and symptoms based on mass effect, but the subdural empyema produces mass effect as well as direct irritation of the cerebral cortex manifest by seizures and focal deficits not accounted for by mass effect alone. Usually epidural abscess follows trauma, craniotomy, paranasal sinus, or mastoid sinus infections. Subdural empyema commonly follows meningitis in infants, but may also follow paranasal sinusitis.

Staphylococcal infections account for most traumatic and post-craniotomy causes of epidural as well as subdural empyema. Those associated with sinus infections reflect the organism found in the sinuses: aerobic and anaerobic streptococci and *Staphylococcus aureus*. Similarly, following meningitis in infants *Haemophilus influenzae* and *Streptococcus pneumoniae* are common causes of subdural empyema.

Clinically, the two entities are distinct: epidural abscess presents with mild symptomatology — a low-grade fever, modest nuchal rigidity, headache and a subgaleal swollen area that is mildly tender and erythematous. In contrast patients with subdural empyema are usually seriously ill and represent a neurosurgical emergency. They are febrile, complain of headache, and have distinct nuchal rigidity. Seizures occur in more than half of these cases. The CT scan aids in the diagnosis of both types of extra-axial infection. Epidural abscesses are usually obvious as extra-axial lucencies,but subdural empyema may present with only subtle findings on CT scan. LP is potentially very dangerous in a patient with mass effect on CT scan, and should therefore be avoided. In the past, however, CSF results have shown normal sugar, elevated protein, a mild pleocytosis and usually a negative culture. Treatment involves drainage of the infection, the removal of adjacent devascularised bone, and the appropriate antibiotics. Patients with epidural abscess usually do well, but there is a 25% mortality and morbidity for patients with subdural empyema.

## Spinal sites

Spinal epidural abscess represents a rare but important clinical entity. Early recognition is critical in preserving neurological function. Approximately two-thirds of all cases evolve over a period of hours to several days. The remainder present indolently over weeks to months. Clinically pain is the rule. It is excruciating and well localised. A palpably tender area can usually be identified posteriorly in the midline, and there is often associated radicular pain. Radicular sensory loss or bowel and bladder dysfunction can be presenting symptoms. Systemic evidence for infection may also be evident. The usual cause is bacteraemia from a distant source (urinary tract or furuncles most commonly). In one-third of cases there is no history of antecedent infection on contamination. Concurrent spinal involvement by the infection may complicate the situation with vertebral body collapse or disc protrusion. The neurological deficits reflect the area of adjacent spinal cord or spinal nerves affected and can progress rapidly to complete spinal cord dysfunction. Almost all patients will demonstrate a complete block on Queckenstedt's manoeuvre. Lumbar puncture should be delayed until myelography can be performed. If abscess fluid is identified epidurally during the lumbar puncture, the needle should not be advanced intradurally, so as to prevent intradural spread of the infection. CSF studies reveal an increased white blood cell count. The predominant cell type is indicative of the type of organism; chemistries show a normal glucose and an elevated protein. Organisms are not typically cultured from CSF. The myelogram reveals epidural compression. Half of the cases result from haematogenous spread of infection and the rest by direct extension from adjacent lesions. Although osteomyelitis is uncommon in an acute epidural empyema, it is seen in approximately one-half of chronic cases. The most frequent organism found in acute epidural abscess is *Staphylococcus aureus*. Other organisms include

*Streptococcus pneumoniae*, other streptococci and *Pseudomonas*. Tuberculosis is the most frequent cause of chronic epidural abscess.

The usual treatment is urgent drainage and subsequent initiation of appropriate antibiotics. A penicillinase-resistant penicillin and an aminoglycoside are recommended for acute epidural abscess. This combination treats both staphylococcal and streptococcal infections as well as many gram-negative rods. Isoniazid, rifampicin and ethambutol are used for tuberculosis, and amphotericin B for most fungal infections. Since outcome reflects the pre-operative neurological deficit and the timing of operative decompression, every effort should be made to diagnose the condition as early as possible.

Spinal subdural empyemas are rare. They result from infected dermal sinuses or concurrent spinal epidural abscess. Presenting signs and symptoms are similar to epidural infection, but pain may be entirely absent. Treatment is similar to epidural abscess, with intradural drainage and the use of appropriate antibiotics.


## OSTEOMYELITIS

### Skull

Osteomyelitis of the skull is uncommon. Its causes are trauma or adjacent infection (usually from frontal sinusitis). The clinical course can be acute or chronic. The acute picture is usually associated with frontal sinusitis resulting in frontal osteomyelitis. The course involves focal pain, pyrexia, and tenderness (Pott's, puffy tumour). The associated bony destruction takes up to 2 weeks to become radiologically evident. The most common organism found is *Staphylococcus aureus* although anaerobic organisms are also known to cause this infection. It is often cultured from direct aspiration or bone biopsy. Treatment should focus on surgical debridement of the involved bone and use of a penicillinase-resistant penicillin until an organism can be implicated. Initial treatment includes IV antibiotics, but after 1 to 2 weeks oral antibiotics capable of producing adequate blood levels are often used.


### Spine

Osteomyelitis of the spine may be difficult to diagnose because of its insidious onset. Patients' complaints include localised pain, weight loss, and, less reliably, intermittent fever. Most commonly there are muscle spasms and limitation of movement. Neurological signs and symptoms occur in only one-quarter of cases and are delayed. These related to vertebral collapse or herniation of disc and bone fragments. The route of infection is usually haematogenous from a distant site such as urinary tract infection, a long-standing abscess or an operative procedure. Direct extension of a contiguous abscess also produces this syndrome.

The white blood cell count and the sedimentation rate are not uniformly elevated. However, serum alkaline phosphatase is usually raised. Blood cultures are positive in 50% of the cases more frequently for *Staphylococcus aureus*. Other organisms include *E. coli* and *Pseudomonas*. Mycobacterial osteomyelitis is common only where tuberculosis persists.

X-rays are initially normal, with the onset of demonstrable changes after 8–12 weeks. Technetium bone scanning is a sensitive early method of localising the infectious site. The CT myelogram is also helpful in evaluating for a paraspinal abscess and spinal canal involvement. Treatment should begin only after identification of the organism. This can be done by blood culture but may require closed or open biopsy. Treatment includes institution of effective antibiotics and spinal stabilisation. This usually involves simple bracing or surgery with bone grafting and fusion. The extent and timing of this surgery depends on the degree of bone destruction. For patients with spinal cord compromise, the prognosis for return of neurological function depends on the severity of neurological impairment prior to operative decompression and stabilisation.

## VIRAL ENCEPHALITIS

Viral encephalitis is the most serious of the viral infections of the central nervous system. These syndromes are characterised by systemic findings of infection such as fever, malaise and headache. Neurological signs may be generalised such as delirium, stupor, coma and seizures, or there may be specific focal neurological dysfunction. The latter takes the form of hemiparesis, sensory deficit, hemianopsia, speech disorder or brainstem dysfunction. These signs are frequently accompanied by a CSF leucocytosis (predominantly monocytes), a mild CSF protein elevation and a normal glucose. Epidemiologically encephalitis falls into two main categories: sporadic and epidemic. The former includes the infections caused by respiratory and enteric viruses. The latter is made up of arthropod-borne infections with togaviruses representing a large proportion.

## Herpes simplex encephalitis

The most common form of fatal sporadic encephalitis is herpes simplex encephalitis. In the United States this accounts for approximately 1000–2000 cases per year or 5–10% of the total cases of encephalitis. Untreated, this infection has a case fatality ratio of at least 70%. Fortunately, there are two efficacious antiviral agents: adenosine arabinoside and acyclovir. The latter appears to be the drug of choice. It is activated by viral thymidine kinase, but not host thymidine kinase. Thus activation only occurs in cells where the herpes simplex virus (HSV) is replicating. Subsequently, DNA transcription is inhibited. Because of this selective activation, acyclovir is 10 times more potent as a inhibitor of HSV DNA replication than of human DNA replication. Because acyclovir appears to be of significant benefit for patients, an imperative exists for clinicians: the early recognition and treatment of HSV encephalitis. For the clinician faced with a probable case of encephalitis, the early diagnosis and treatment of HSV encephalitis gives those patients a significant chance of a normal recovery from an otherwise fatal illness.

Herpes simplex encephalitis characteristically presents with an inferior temporal and temporo-frontal focus. This localisation occurs uniformly on autopsy specimens. It has been postulated that it represents reactivation of latent virus from the Gasserian ganglion. The clinical presentation is of a medial temporal lesion. Systemic symptoms of fever and headache progress to a hemiparesis, aphasia and obtundation over about 7 days. Seizures occur in up to half of the patients. EEG, brain scan and CT frequently show a focal abnormality in the medial portion of the temporal lobe. However, early infections do not produce obvious abnormalities, particularly on CT. Unfortunately, many other infectious processes can randomly present with a medial temporal localisation. Thus, over 20% of the patients in a recent study were diagnosed as having a non-herpetic cerebral infection by brain biopsy. One-half of these individuals had bacterial, fungal, tubercular or toxoplasma abscesses requiring a different specific antibiotic therapy. Biopsy of inferior temporal lesions is necessary to properly define the aetiology and treatment

129

of these processes. In our cooperative study, biopsy was safe with no mortality and 2% morbidity. The mortality of treated HSV encephalitis in a recent multicentre study was 35%. No mortality occurred for individuals under 30 who were conscious when acyclovir was administered. Of this group 50% had no disability on follow-up examination and were able to return to their previous occupations.

## Other viral encephalitides

Other viruses account for about 90% of the cases of encephalitis. These viruses include the enteroviruses, mumps, cytomegalovirus, lymphocytic choriomeningitis and the togaviruses. These agents are difficult to distinguish clinically since fever, seizures and altered mental state usually dominate the clinical picture. The prodromal illness and associated organ involved can provide helpful clues. Enterovirus encephalitis frequently has a prodromal diarrhoea/illness with accompanying pleural, pericardial, myocardial and/or enteric inflammation, and mumps can be associated with parotitis, pancreatitis and/or orchitis. The case fatality ratio of these agents is less than 10%. However, the arthropod-borne viruses may have a ratio closer to 25%. In North America these togavirus infections are likely to be mosquito borne and caused by the eastern and western equine encephalitis viruses. In Europe they would be tick-borne and produce central European or Russian spring–summer encephalitis.

The other viral infection that can present as an encephalitic syndrome is rabies. Here a case-fatality ratio close to one is seen. Diagnostically a history of an antecedent animal bite (weeks prior) is often given. This infection is much more frequent among citizens of and travellers to underdeveloped countries, but epidemic zoonosis can occur throughout the world with spread to the local human population based on contact with the infected animal species.

There are no specific therapies of prove efficacy for these viral encephalitides. Acyclovir has *in vitro* activity against varicella-zoster virus and vidarabine against cytomegalovirus, but the clinical value of this potential efficacy has not yet been established. General therapeutic measures for encephalitis victims should include anticonvulsant therapy, nutritional support and close observation with sedation and restraints. Cerebral oedema can be associated with intracranial hypertension; therefore, judicious fluid restriction and occasional monitoring of intracranial pressure are probably helpful in these situations. Elevated intracranial pressure should be identified and treated when the patient has ongoing status epilepticus. In these patients and other comatose patients with impaired airway reflexes, endotracheal intubation should be performed to prevent aspiration and assist in clearing secretions.

## BRAIN ABSCESS

Brain abscess usually presents as a focal deficit. Fever and elevated white blood cell count occur in only about 50% of the cases. There are two main mechanisms of infection: direct spread of bacteria from an adjacent cranial site or haematogenous spread. The nasal and mastoid sinuses are the most common sources for direct extension of infection. Bacterial endocarditis, pulmonary abscess, bronchiectasis, or right to left cardiac shunts are the major antecedents to haematogenous spread. Immunocompromised patients and intravenous drug abusers have frequent bacteraemias and are at significant risk for brain abscess. Lumbar puncture should be avoided, if brain abscess is suspected, but the CSF is frequently sterile with a pleocytosis, elevated protein and a normal glucose. EEG and radionuclide brain scan can be used to confirm the localisation of a focal deficit. CT usually demonstrates a lucency with mass effect; contrast produces uniform enhancement during early stages and a ring enhancement later as the abscess matures.

Initial clinical efforts should be made to define the primary source of the infection, the extent of non-cerebral involvement, and most importantly the identification of the causative organism. For this reason we strongly advocate early surgical drainage of cerebral abscesses. This is the most direct method for identifying the pathogen, and is done by craniotomy and excision of an encapsulated mass, direct needle aspiration or stereotactic aspiration. The latter method is the technique of choice for brainstem and other deep lesions not amenable to open surgery. The surgical approach allows for optimal drainage and identification of the causative organism prior to the start of antibiotics. *Staphylococcus aureus, Streptococcus viridans* and less frequently anaerobic and gram-negative bacteria are cultured from the abscess cavity. Initial antibiotic therapy should reflect the likely organism for the clinical setting of each patient. A penicillinase-resistant penicillin for staphylococci and chloramphenicol for anaerobic bacterial coverage are frequently

131

the initial post-operative antibiotics chosen. Antibiotic treatment should be altered on the basis of bacterial identification and subsequent susceptibility testing. Optimal dosing schedules can be determined by assessment of serum bacteriocidal activity. This is of particular importance when bacterial endocarditis has been diagnosed. Usually treatment is given intravenously for 4 to 6 weeks. Seizures are the most common complication, occurring acutely in about 25% of the cases. Anticonvulsant prophylaxis with phenytoin or phenobarbital should be part of the treatment regimen. Rupture with ventriculitis and meningitis can be a life-threatening complication. This is best avoided by adequate initial drainage, optimal antibiotic coverage based on *in vitro* sensitivity testing and frequent follow-up CT assessments. Reaccumulation of abscess fluid calls for a repeat drainage procedure usually via the stereotactic approach. Overall, mortality is still in the 30–40% range, with younger patients more likely to survive.

**FURTHER READING**

Britt, R.H. (1985) Brain abscess. In: R.H. Wilkins and S.S. Rengachany *Neurosurgery*, McGraw Hill, New York, pp. 1928–1956
Johnson, E.T. (1982) *Viral infections of the nervous system*, Raven Press, New York
Sande, M.A., Smith, A.L. and Root, R.K. (1985) *Bacterial meningitis*, Churchill Livingstone, New York
Spetzler, R.F. and Zabramski, J.M. (1986) Cerebrospinal fluid fistula *Contemp. Neurosurg.* 8(1), 1–8
Whitley, R.A. *et al.* (1986) Herpes simplex encephalitis: adenine arabinoside versus acyclovir therapy. *New Engl. J. Med. 314*, 144–9
Youmans, J.R. (1982) *Neurological surgery*, W.B. Saunders, Philadelphia

# 8

## Acute Intoxications

Russell J.M. Lane and Peter G. Blain

**INTRODUCTION**

Each year more than 100 000 people are admitted to British hospitals as a result of deliberate or accidental poisoning. The major insult under such circumstances is frequently to the central nervous system. Neurological disorders due to intoxications may arise in two other circumstances: as an adverse drug reaction or drug interaction, and as a result of accidental exposure to chemicals at work or at home, usually from inhalation of vapours or penetration through the skin. Add to these the increasing problems of alcohol and street drug abuse and it is clear that neurological disturbances resulting from acute intoxications are relatively common problems in medical practice. The purpose of this chapter is to describe the types of neurological disorder which can arise under such circumstances, to indicate any features which should suggest that a neurological disorder is drug- or chemically induced and, where appropriate, to outline specific measures which might be undertaken as first lines of treatment. Examples of drugs and chemicals that are commonly implicated will be given, but for further information the reader is referred to the more comprehensive reviews listed at the end of this chapter.

**GENERAL POINTS ON MANAGEMENT**

The nature of the drugs or chemicals responsible for an acute intoxication may not be immediately clear. Indeed, in self-poisoning the patient not infrequently takes a mixture of drugs, often with alcohol. Immediate management is therefore directed to general supportive measures, notably careful maintenance of the airway, assisted ventilation by Ambu bag and oxygen where necessary, and management of hypotension, hypothermia, cardiac dysrhythmias and seizures. Any patient showing even mild features of neurological dysfunction should be admitted to hospital, particularly if drugs with a delayed action, such as tricyclic antidepressants, are involved. If the patient is conscious and cooperative, and the ingested poison is not a corrosive or petroleum distillate, it is worth attempting to empty the stomach by giving ipecacuanha emetic mixture (30 ml in adults, 10–15 ml in children). If vomiting is not persistent, this might be followed by an activated charcoal preparation (Carbomix or Medicoal, 50–100 g in water) prior to transport to hospital.

It is worth emphasising at the outset that nearly all neurological disorders due to acute intoxications are completely reversible with appropriate conservative management. Few specific antidotes are available, and careful control of fluid balance and avoidance of metabolic acidosis and hypokalaemia are paramount. Techniques such as forced diuresis, haemodialysis and charcoal haemoperfusion are of value in severe cases of poisoning with certain agents but will not be discussed here.

Adverse drug reactions are of two types. *Type A (augmented) reactions* are an exaggeration of normal pharmacological actions. They are dose-dependent and thus easily identified. *Type B (idiosyncratic) reactions* are *qualitatively* abnormal, inexplicable in terms of the known pharmacology of the drug and may involve immunological mechanisms. Morbidity and mortality from such effects are higher since they are unpredictable, and at best one can hope for early detection and discontinuation of the drug.

It is convenient to consider the neurology of acute intoxications in terms of site of involvement and clinical presentation (Table 8.1).

## CEREBRAL CORTEX

### Coma

Coma and lesser changes in conscious level generally result from one of three mechanisms: primary effects on the nervous system, indirect effects on cerebral metabolism and alterations in cerebral blood flow (Table 8.2).

*Drug-induced coma* is most commonly due to overdosage with *neuroleptics* such as the benzodiazepines, phenothiazines,

**Table 8.1**: Neurological disorders due to acute intoxications

| | |
|---|---|
| *Cerebral cortex:* | *Disorders of voluntary movement:* |
| Coma | Tremor |
| Neuropsychiatric effects | Acute dystonia |
| Seizures | Chorea and athetosis |
| Strokes | Dyskinesias |
| *Headache and intracranial* | Neuroleptic malignant syndrome |
| *hypertension* | *Neuromuscular disorders:* |
| *Visual symptoms and deafness* | Peripheral neuropathies |
| *Ataxia* | Myasthenia |
| | Myopathies |
| | Myotonia |

**Table 8.2**: Drugs and chemicals associated with seizures

| | |
|---|---|
| *Analgesics* | *Antidepressants* |
| Cocaine | Amitryptiline |
| Pethidine | Imipramine |
| Dextropropoxyphene | MAOIs |
| | Viloxazine |
| *Anticonvulsants* | |
| Valproate | *Hormones* |
| | Glucocorticoids |
| *Antiarrythmics* | Insulin |
| Disopyramide | Oxytocin |
| Lignocaine | Prostaglandins |
| | |
| *Antibacterials* | *Phenothiazines* |
| Penicillins | Chlorpromazine |
| Cephalosporins | Prochlorpromazine |
| Isoniazid | Promazine |
| Nalidixic acid | |
| | *Respiratory stimulants* |
| *Chemicals* | Amiphenazole |
| Organic solvents | Doxapram |
| Petroleum distillates | |
| Metaldehyde | *Bronchodilators* |
| Glycol | Terbutaline |
| | Theophylline |
| *Miscellaneous* | Salbutamol |
| Factor VIII | |
| Lithium | *Anti-inflammatory analgesics* |
| Pyrimethamine | Mefenamic acid |
| Vincristine | |
| Thallium | |
| Cyclosporin | |

antidepressants, lithium, barbiturates and narcotics. Severe poisoning with many industrial and household chemicals can also result in coma, frequently associated with seizures and myoclonus. Examples include metaldehyde (in slug pellets), phenoxyacetate herbicides such as Mecoprop, petroleum distillates (turpentine substitute, white spirit, liquid polishes), organic solvents, methanol and ethylene glycol. Other groups of drugs such as $\beta$-blockers and diuretics have occasionally been implicated. The last decade has seen a reduction in the incidence of overdose with drugs such as methaqualone, barbiturates and the first-generation benzodiazepines, and an increase in poisoning with antidepressants and newer minor tranquillisers such as flurazepam, which can produce a prolonged coma.

*Coma due to metabolic disturbances* can occur with drugs in therapeutic doses as well as overdosage. Hypoglycaemic coma due to insulin and oral hypoglycaemic agents may be preceded by behavioural abnormalities and seizures. Sulphonylureas particularly can produce a profound hypoglycaemia which is remarkably refractory to intravenous glucose and may be complicated by hyponatraemia secondary to stimulation of ADH secretion. Methanol intoxication is classically associated with visual disturbances due to optic nerve damage by formaldehyde and other metabolites. Symptoms include changes in colour perceptions and constriction of the visual fields, progressing to total blindness. Features of general intoxication may include dizziness, headache, diplopia and behavioural disturbances, leading to coma and death if poisoning is severe. A severe metabolic acidosis with a large anion gap is characteristic.

Sudden changes in cerebral blood flow can produce syncope and sometimes coma. *Vasodilators* such as glyceryl trinitrate, prazocin and calcium antagonists (verapamil, nifedipine) may cause collapse of peripheral resistance, with flushing, headache, tachycardia, hypotension and syncope. Similar symptoms may also occur in *postural hypotension*, which may be a complication of treatment with several antihypertensives (such as bethanidine, debrisoquine, guanethidine, clonidine) with most of the monoamine oxidase inhibitors (MAOIs) and tricyclic antidepressants.

*Strokes* resulting in coma and other severe neurological disorders, can also be drug-induced. Examples include cerebral arterial and venous thrombosis associated with use of oral contraceptives, and cerebral haemorrhage as a result of hypertension induced by sympathomimetic amines (for example in the tyramine 'cheese' reaction with MAOIs) or as a result of overdosage with anticoagulants.

The clinical features of drug-induced coma are generally similar regardless of the drug involved. Typically, the pupillary and corneal reflexes are preserved while other brainstem reflexes (e.g. the doll's eye and gag reflexes) are impaired at an early stage. Tone in the limbs is usually markedly reduced, the tendon reflexes are depressed or absent and the plantar responses are flexor or equivocal. In cases of tricyclic overdosage and hepatic coma, and exceptionally with other intoxications, hyper-reflexia and extensor plantar responses may be found and myoclonus and seizures may occur. Coma due to opiates typically produces pin-point pupils and it may be necessary to use a hand lens to assess the pupillary responses, whereas with tricyclic overdose the pupils are often widely dilated. In deep coma all reflexes may be lost; indeed, the neurological features of brainstem death may be present. Coma due to drugs, chemicals and metabolic disturbances must be excluded before making such a diagnosis.

The management of drug-induced coma is essentially supportive with particular attention to protection of the airway, since vomiting and aspiration pneumonia are the main life-threatening complications in this situation. Specific treatment is rarely possible. When opiate overdosage is suspected, it is essential to give emergency treatment with intravenous naloxone 0.8–2.0 mg every 2–3 minutes until the patient responds. The effect is short-lived, however, and a continuous infusion may be required. It can be dramatic, with rapid recovery of consciousness. Physostigmine can reverse the anti-cholinergic effects of antidepressants and improve conscious level but the effects are short-lived and this drug can cause vomiting, bronchial hypersecretion, seizures and cardiac dysrhythmias and is not recommended. Methanol produces its toxic effects by oxidation to formaldehyde and formic acid. This can be competitively inhibited by ethanol, and an intravenous infusion of 10–15 g per hour, possibly with folinic acid 30 mg intravenously every 6 hours to limit ocular toxicity, should be given.


### Neuropsychiatric effects

The commonest drug involved in overdosage is of course *alcohol*. The general effects of ethanol intoxication are well known but it must always be borne in mind that patients who simply appear drunk may have taken other drugs or have sustained head injuries. Alcoholic poisoning may be complicated by hypoglycaemia and lactic acidosis, and the development of confusion and confabulation, with nystagmus and ataxia, in an alcoholic should suggest the possibility of Wernicke's encephalopathy, requiring urgent treatment with thiamin.

Psychomotor performance will be impaired by any of the *neuroleptics* or other drugs which can precipitate coma, and by overexposure to the vapour of many industrial *solvents* with properties similar to anaesthetic gases, such as trichlorethylene, perchlorethylene, carbon tetrachloride, toluene and xylene. The craze of 'glue-sniffing', now referred to as 'volatile substance abuse' since other substances such as lighter fuel, polishes and aerosols may be involved, can also result in an acute confusional state with hallucinations and excitation leading to coma and metabolic acidosis. Mild carbon monoxide poising can also cause a confusional state, with headache, nausea and malaise. n-Hexane and acrylamide vapours produce increasing drowsiness, dizziness, nausea and ataxia. Chronic exposure to all these chemicals may produce an axonal polyneuropathy.

## Seizures

Acute intoxication with drugs and chemicals may occasionally result in seizures. Although many drugs have been reported to induce seizures, there is actually little evidence of direct implication in most cases. Compounds for which evidence of convulsive action is much stronger are listed in Table 8.2.

Drug-induced seizures are clinically indistinguishable from those due to other causes. Generalised motor seizures occur most commonly but partial seizures may also develop. Patients with established epilepsy or known cerebral disease are most vulnerable, but drugs may precipitate seizures in apparently healthy individuals, particularly when there is a family history of epilepsy.

Compounds most often involved are those that are given for their *direct effects on the CNS*, such as antipsychotics, antidepressants and analgesics. These readily cross the blood–brain barrier, and seizures are most likely to occur with large doses of drug, or where *renal* or *hepatic insufficiency* results in high plasma drug concentrations (Type A reaction). Seizures may follow poisoning with a wide range of other drugs and chemicals including $\beta_2$-adrenoreceptor agonists, methyl xanthines, anti-inflammatory drugs such as mefenamic acid, various herbicides and insecticides such as pyrethroids, organophosphates, petroleum distillates, alcohols, and glycols. Seizures and other neurological problems such as coma, ataxia, tremor and myclonus have also been reported with cyclosporin.

Certain compounds within a class of drug may be more prone to induce seizures than others and this may influence choice of treatment. For example, phenothiazines with an aliphatic side-chain (chlorpromazine, prochlorperazine, promazine) are more epileptogenic than those with a piperazine side-chain (fluphenazine, trifluoperazine). Similarly, terbutaline may be preferred to theophylline in reversible airways disease, and although all antidepressants lower the seizure threshold, mianserin and nomifensine may be safer than imipramine and amitryptiline in patients at risk.

Drugs may cause seizures in three other circumstances. Certain *drug interactions* may produce or exacerbate seizures. For example, the conversion of pethidine to nor-pethidine, which has greater epileptogenic potential but less analgesic effect than the parent drug, is increased by phenobarbitone through hepatic enzyme induction, and administration of pethidine to patients on MAOIs is contraindicated as this may result in convulsions, delirium and hyperpyrexia.

*Rapid changes in plasma concentration* of drugs which are cerebral irritants in high concentration may induce seizures. Examples include intravenous lignocaine for the treatment of cardiac dysrhythmias after myocardial infarction, theophylline and terbutaline for acute bronchospasm, and even penicillin and its derivatives, particularly if renal insufficiency is present.

Thirdly, some drugs may predispose to seizures indirectly by causing *changes in intermediary metabolism*. Hypoglycaemia due to insulin and oral hypoglycaemics has already been mentioned, and isoniazid and cycloserine may occasionally cause seizures, particularly in slow acetylators, possibly by causing cerebral pyridoxine deficiency. Very rarely, seizures can follow vaccination, for example with pertussis or measles, presumably through an immunological mechanism, although this appears to be far more likely to occur in infants with brain damage or who have suffered seizures previously.

Paradoxically, the commonest cause of drug-related seizures is *drug withdrawal*. Non-compliance with anticonvulsant medication and abrupt discontinuation of habituating drugs such as ethanol, barbiturates and benzodiazepines are the usual causes. Seizures may also be a feature of *poisoning* with a number of chemicals including thallium, strychnine and carbon monoxide.

The management of seizures in the context of poisoning differs slightly from that employed in an epileptic, or for seizures arising as a result of structural brain damage or inflammation, since the convulsions are a manifestation of intoxication and are unlikely to recur after recovery. Repeated doses of diazepam (intravenously *not* intramuscularly) or a chlormethiazole infusion should be employed and anticonvulsants avoided if possible.

## Drug-induced headache

Drugs can occasionally precipitate severe headache. In general, this results from stretching of the pain-sensitive blood vessels or meninges. Compounds which produce headache as a result of *vasodilatation* include glyceryl trinitrate, hydrallazine, nifedipine, perhexilene, theophylline and terbutaline. Headache can also be caused by *vasoconstrictors* such as bromocriptine or by acute withdrawal of vasoactive compounds such as caffeine, ergotamine and methysergide. *Sudden changes in blood pressure*, as with the introduction or sudden withdrawal of clonidine, prazosin and β-adrenoreceptor blockers, may also precipitate headache.

Drugs can also produce headache by *stretching or irritation of the meninges*. Indomethacin and other non-steroidal anti-inflammatory drugs may cause changes in intra- and extravascular fluid volume due to their salt- and water-retaining properties, and a number of unrelated compounds have been associated with the development of benign intracranial hypertension (pseudotumour cerebri, Table 8.3). There are also reports of patients developing an aseptic meningitis while taking sulindac, tolmetin, ibuprofen and co-trimoxazole.

Clinical features are of little value in differentiating drug-induced headache from other potentially more serious causes. The temporal relationship of headache to drug administration may be of value when vasoactive drugs are involved, and the development of headache with papilloedema (and rarely non-localising cranial nerve pareses) in a young woman taking an appropriate medication should suggest a diagnosis of drug-induced intracranial hypertension. Headache due to digoxin and theophylline may be prevented by monitoring plasma concentrations.

## Visual symptoms and deafness

Rarely, acute intoxications can cause impairment of visual acuity

**Table 8.3:** Drugs causing intracranial hypertension

| | |
|---|---|
| Nalidixic acid | Steroids |
| Nitrofurantoin | Perhexilene |
| Nitrous oxide | Tetracyclines |
| Vitamin A | |

**Table 8.4:** Oculo- and ototoxic drugs

| Visual symptoms | Deafness |
|---|---|
| *Anti-inflammatory drugs* | *Antibiotics* |
| Ibuprofen | Gentamicin |
| Indomethacin | Tobramycin |
| Salicylates | Chloramphenicol |
| | Erythromycin |
| *Antimicrobials* | |
| Ethambutol | *Diuretics* |
| Chloroquine | Ethacrynic acid |
| Quinine | Bumetanide |
| | Frusemide |
| *Miscellaneous* | |
| Chlorpropamide | *Miscellaneous* |
| Digoxin | Aspirin |
| Oral contraceptives | Indomethacin |
| Penicillamine | Propranolol |

and even frank blindness, by damaging the retina or optic nerves (Table 8.4). *Dyschromatopsia* has been reported with a number of drugs and is a notable early feature of digoxin toxicity. Diuretics have been implicated as a cause of *acute visual failure* due to central retinal oedema and macular swelling. *Retinal vascular disorders* can be caused by several types of drug. For example, oral contraceptives can precipitate retinal artery occlusion or retinal vein thrombosis, and scotomas due to retinal haemorrhages have been reported in association with anti-inflammatory analgesics and sulphonamides. Quinine poisoning may cause acute retinal vasospasm, resulting in visual blurring which may progress to complete blindness. Fixed dilated pupils, papilloedema and retinal oedema may occur and may be followed by optic atrophy and persistent tunnel vision. Acute *optic neuritis* may be caused by several types of antimicrobials, notably the antituberculous drugs. Optic neuropathy is also a prominent feature of methanol poisoning. Visual cortical damage producing *cortical blindness* can succeed severe hypotension following poisoning with several types of drug, including salicylates, barbiturates and chloral hydrate, and has been reported following routine treatment with capreomycin, nalidixic acid and bromocriptine.

Several groups of drugs are potentially ototoxic and can damage both cochlear and vestibular structures (Table 8.4). *Drug-induced deafness* often develops insidiously and the patient may be unaware of the problem until a precipitous fall in auditory acuity occurs. Occasionally ototoxic effects may be more acute, heralded by tinnitus or accompanied by features of vestibular toxicity such as vertigo, ataxia and nausea, with nystagmus. Drug-induced ototoxicity is nearly always a dose-related (Type A) adverse effect, and patients with renal insufficiency or pre-existing sensorineural deafness are particularly at risk. The aminoglycosides and polymixins are most frequently implicated, and the effects of sustained high levels of these drugs are often irreversible. *Diuretics* can occasionally produce acute deafness following intravenous administration, particularly when renal function is impaired. Ethacrynic acid appears to be most toxic in this regard, followed by frusemide and bumetanide, but thiazides have not been implicated. Deafness has also been reported with administration of large doses of aspirin and other *non-steroidal anti-inflammatory drugs*.

**Ataxia**

Intoxication with benzodiazepines, antipsychotic drugs and anticonvulsants can result in signs and symptoms of cerebellar dysfunction with dysarthria, nystagmus and truncal and limb ataxia. Cimetidine has also rarely been reported to produce such symptoms. Again, there are no specific clinical features that will differentiate drug-induced ataxia from other causes, which may have to be excluded by investigation. The increasing availability of serum anticonvulsant measurements should reduce the incidence of drug toxicity in epileptic patients.

**Involuntary movements**

Involuntary movements are among the most dramatic neurological manifestations of acute intoxications, and drugs can reproduce any of the spontaneously occurring movement disorders. Exaggeration of physiological *tremor* can be produced by caffeine, tricyclic antidepressants, anticonvulsants and lithium, and by withdrawal of alcohol, barbiturates and benzodiazepines after chronic use. Severe tremor is also a prominent feature of mercury poisoning. *Asterixis* and *myoclonus* may develop in anticonvulsant toxicity, particularly with sodium valproate.

*Acute dystonia*, an alarming movement disorder most often encountered in children and young adults, has been described following administration of many types of antipsychotic drugs, and also of metaclopramide, tricyclic antidepressants, phenytoin and carbamazepine, and propranolol in high doses. The onset is often abrupt and may be mistaken for hysteria or even tetany. The muscles of the head and neck are mainly affected, with spasm of the tongue, trismus and facial grimacing and other orofacial dyskinesias. Oculogyric crises, torticollis and retrocollis, opisthotonus, axial dystonias and a bizarre gait can occur and are often accompanied by writhing movements of the limbs. The attacks are episodic and, while frightening to witness or experience, are usually painless. Between each episode muscle tone is normal, and during a subsequent attack different muscle groups may be affected. Drug-induced dystonia usually remits in hours to days once the offending drug is withdrawn, but intravenous benztropine or diazepam are useful in severe cases.

*Chorea*, an irregular fine jerking or fidgeting movement of the limbs, which may be accompanied by the slow writhing movements of athetosis, or by dystonia, has been reported in patients taking oral contraceptives; anabolic steroids have also been implicated. The most frequent association has been with antipsychotic drugs and anticonvulsants, especially phenytoin. The effects are not clearly dose related, however, and appear to be a Type B reaction in most cases.

*Dyskinesias* are often encountered in Parkinson's disease in patients taking *L*-dopa preparations, and can develop in both the initial stages of treatment and with chronic treatment. The commonest dyskinesias involve the lips, facial muscles and tongue, but the trunk and limbs can be involved in severe cases. The effects are Type A reactions and usually cease when the dose is reduced.

## Neuroleptic malignant syndrome

This is a rare and potentially fatal reaction most commonly associated with the phenothiazines, thioxanthines and butyrophenones. The pathogenesis is not fully understood but appears to be related to dopamine receptor blockade, including the thermoregulatory and vasomotor centres. It is usually precipitated by initiating or increasing the doses of neuroleptics. Initially there is a rapid and progressive increase in extrapyramidal rigidity and a failure of vasomotor regulation, leading to an increase in body temperature secondary to increasing muscular contraction, although hyperthermia is not invariable. Involuntary movements may occur together with features of autonomic disturbance such as sweating, tachydysrhythmias and labile blood pressure. The patient may become mute, rigid and stuporose, and seizures, coma and death may follow. The serum creatine kinase is usually raised, often to high levels, and there may be biochemical features of dehydration and renal failure, as well as abnormal liver function tests and a leucocytosis. Treatment involves withdrawal of offending drugs and administration of the dopamine agonist bromocriptine and the muscle relaxant dantrolene sodium.

## Neuromuscular disorders

The peripheral nerves, neuromuscular junctions and skeletal muscles can be damaged by a wide range of drugs and chemicals but only a few of these need be considered in the context of acute intoxications.

*Peripheral neuropathies* due to drugs usually develop insidiously over months or years but acute polyneuropathy may occur with nitrofurantoin, isoniazid and other antituberculous drugs, and with most cytotoxics, notably vincristine. Perhexilene maleate and amiodarone can produce a similar problem. Typically the clinical features are of a symmetrical sensorimotor polyneuropathy, with a 'glove and stocking' sensory loss, areflexia and variable degrees of mainly distal weakness.

Predominantly motor polyneuropathy may be seen with sulphonamides, tricyclic antidepressants, cimetidine and indomethacin. Lead intoxication causes a motor neuropathy which in adults particularly affects the extensors of the wrists and occasionally the feet; intoxication in children leads to an encephalopathy.

Occasionally painful paraesthesiae, proximal weakness and even cranial nerve involvement may develop in drug-induced neuropathies. Previous subclinical damage to nerves, for example by diabetes or ethanol, increases the risk of neuropathy from drugs. Drugs and other poisons generally cause axonal damage, but gold injections have been reported to precipitate a demyelinating polyneuropathy (presenting as a Guillain-Barré syndrome), presumably through an immunological mechanism.

*Neuralgic amyotrophy* (brachial plexus neuritis), characterised by severe pain in the shoulder or arm, followed by rapid wasting of shoulder girdle muscles and sometimes sensory loss over the deltoid region, can follow immunisation or antibiotic injections.

*Mononeuropathies* can be caused by intramuscular injections as a result of direct trauma or haemorrhage, and may result from spontaneous or traumatic haemorrhage around nerves in patients with poorly controlled anticoagulant therapy. *Mononeuritis* and mononeuritis multiplex have followed intra-arterial infusions of cytotoxic agents such as mustine hydrochloride, and have also been reported with intravenous opiate and amphetamine abuse. Symptoms reminiscent of tic douloureux have been described in patients taking digoxin, and trigeminal neuropathy can develop with trichlorethylene and labetolol. The commonest neuropathy following acute intoxication, however, is probably 'Saturday night palsy', neuropraxial damage to the radial nerve after lying on the arm for a long period. Rarely, permanent damage to the peripheral nerves or brachial plexus, or its blood supply, can result from such prolonged compression.

### Myasthenia

Numerous drugs can impair neuromuscular transmission but there is a large inherent safety factor in the mechanism of the normal neuromuscular junction so the effects are usually clinically insignificant. Certain drugs may, however, precipitate a myasthenic crisis, with the dangers of respiratory insufficiency, if the neuromuscular junctions are already damaged. Thus patients with latent myasthenia gravis may develop their first symptoms of exposure to such drugs (Table 8.5). Furthermore, drugs used to treat myasthenia, such as anticholinesterases and steroids, can cause severe weakness and respiratory failure in myasthenic patients if given in large doses.

True myasthenia gravis *precipitated* by drugs is difficult to

145

**Table 8.5:** Drugs which may produce or aggravate myasthenia

| | |
|---|---|
| *Antibiotics* | *Cardiovascular drugs* |
| Aminoglycosides | Lignocaine |
| Clindamycin | Quinidine |
| Lincomycin | Procainamide |
| Tetracycline | Propranolol |
| | |
| *Anticonvulsants* | *Psychotherapeutic drugs* |
| Phenytoin | Lithium |
| | Phenothiazines |
| *Antirheumatic drugs* | |
| Chloroquine | *Hormones* |
| D-penicillamine | Corticosteroids |
| | Thyroid hormone |
| *Anticholinesterases* | |
| Pyridostigmine | |

distinguish on clinical grounds from a *drug-induced myasthenic syndrome*. This only occurs in non-myasthenic individuals when the safety factor for neuromuscular transmission is severely compromised, for example by hypokalaemia or hypocalcaemia. However, D-penicillamine can produce a myasthenic syndrome which is clinically and electrophysiologically identical to myasthenia gravis and which, like the naturally occurring disease, is characterised by the presence of antibodies to the acetylcholine receptor.

Patients with drug-induced myasthenia usually respond to intravenous edrophonium (Tensilon). Subsequent management involves withdrawal of the offending drug and, if symptoms are sufficiently severe, treatment with an anticholinesterase such as prostigmine or pyridostigmine until resolution occurs.

Finally, poisoning with organophosphate and carbamate insecticides inactivates cholinesterases leading to conduction block at the myoneural junction, and in the CNS and autonomic nervous system. This leads to muscle twitching, visual blurring, sweating, salivation, lacrymation and convulsions. The muscarinic effects can be blocked with atropine, and pralidoxine can be given to specifically reactivate the cholinesterases.

## Myopathies

Acute intoxications can sometimes result in severe muscle damage.

The most serious condition which can result is *rhabdomyolysis*, in which there is extensive damage to large numbers of muscle fibres, leading to leakage of intracellular constituents, including enzymes such as creatine kinase, and of myoglobin, potassium and phosphate. This can lead to acute renal failure, serious cardiac dysrhythmias, seizures and coma. Acute rhabdomyolysis is most often associated with ethanol, opiates and other 'street' drugs such as phencyclidine and amphetamines, but can also develop simply as a result of tissue compression in a comatose patient left lying on a hard surface for a long period. The onset is acute with severe muscle pain, tenderness and sometimes marked muscle swelling. There is generalised weakness, more marked proximally than distally, and depressed or absent reflexes. Treatment involves removing the offending drug and careful monitoring of renal function and serum calcium, potassium and phosphate concentration. An infusion of mannitol may help renal function but peritoneal dialysis may be required.

Less severe degrees of intoxication with these drugs, and others, can result in an acute or sub-acute painful proximal myopathy. This may be a necrotising myopathy, caused by direct toxic action on the muscle, or an *inflammatory* myopathy, involving immunological mechanisms, and may rarely result from severe drug-induced *hypokalaemia*. Differentiation of these disorders requires detailed electromyography and muscle biopsy.

*Myotonia* is a rare manifestation of acute intoxication. Propranolol, pindolol, barbiturates and fenterol can aggravate or unmask a pre-existing myotonic disorder, and the muscle cramps associated with certain diuretics may be due to induction of a subclinical myotonia. Myotonia may also be a feature of poisoning with chlorophenoxyacetate herbicides, such as 2,4-dichlorophenoxylate (2,4-D).

## CONCLUSION

The consequences of an acute intoxication are usually reversible provided the cause is recognised sufficiently early. Increasing drug prescription, the development of newer and more powerful drugs, and the growing burden of hazardous chemicals in the environment suggest that we are likely to encounter the neurological complications of acute intoxication with increasing frequency in the future.

## FURTHER READING

Blain, P.G. and Lane, R.J.M. (1983) Drugs and muscle. *Adv. Drug React. Ac. Pois. Rev.* 2, 1–24

Blain, P.G. and Steward-Wynne, E. (1986) Neurological disorders. In: D.M. Davies (ed.) *Textbook of adverse drug reactions*, Oxford University Press, Oxford, pp. 494–514

Lane, R.J.M. and Routledge, P.A. (1983) Drug-induced neurological disorders. *Drugs*, 26, 124–47

# 9

# Respiratory Failure of Neurological Origin

Michael S. Aldrich and Thomas K. Aldrich

## INTRODUCTION

Respiratory failure is probably the most serious complication of neurological diseases. In patients with brainstem dysfunction from tumours, strokes and intracerebral haemorrhages, loss of respiratory drive is a serious threat to life. Respiratory failure due to respiratory muscle weakness and associated complications accounts for the majority of deaths from Duchenne muscular dystrophy (Gilroy *et al.*, 1963; Inkley *et al.*, 1974) and amyotrophic lateral sclerosis (motor neurone disease), and it is an important contributor to morbidity and mortality in spinal cord injuries, myasthenia gravis, and Guillain-Barré syndrome.

Any neurological illness that affects the brainstem, cervical nerve roots, peripheral nerves, neuromuscular junction or proximal muscles can lead to acute or chronic respiratory failure. In this chapter, we will first review the neurological mechanisms that can lead to respiratory failure. We will then discuss the signs and symptoms of respiratory failure and various methods to facilitate diagnosis. We will close with a discussion of therapy and prevention of respiratory failure in these patients.

## MECHANISMS OF IMPAIRMENT

### Pathways of respiratory control

The respiratory system includes two separate but related components: the lungs, which provide for gas exchange, and the ventilatory pump, which provides ventilation to the lungs (Figure 9.1). Since

**Figure 9.1:** Gas exchange failure is due to disorders that affect lung function. Ventilatory failure is due to disorders that affect respiratory drive or impair the ability of the neuromuscular elements of the chest wall and the airways to perform the work of breathing

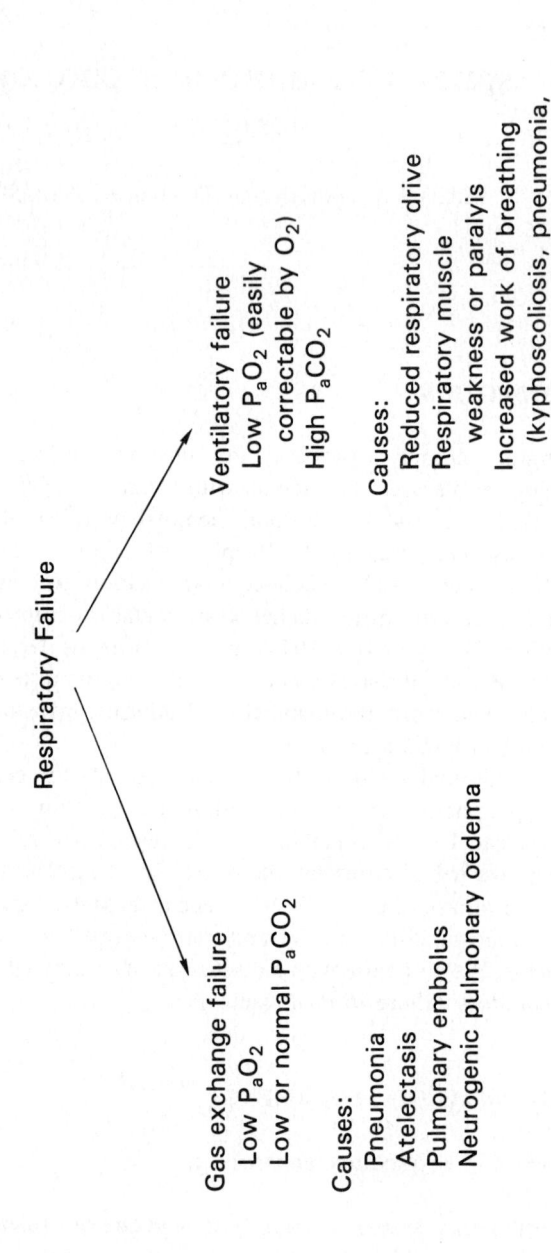

Respiratory Failure

Gas exchange failure
Low $P_aO_2$
Low or normal $P_aCO_2$

Causes:
Pneumonia
Atelectasis
Pulmonary embolus
Neurogenic pulmonary oedema

Ventilatory failure
Low $P_aO_2$ (easily
  correctable by $O_2$)
High $P_aCO_2$

Causes:
Reduced respiratory drive
Respiratory muscle
  weakness or paralyis
Increased work of breathing
  (kyphoscoliosis, pneumonia,
  atelectasis, etc.)

failure of the gas exchange function generally affects the exchange of oxygen more than it affects the exchange of carbon dioxide, it is characterised by hypoxaemia, with little or no carbon dioxide retention in most cases. In contrast, ventilatory failure is characterised primarily by carbon dioxide retention, and the associated mild hypoxaemia is usually easily correctable with supplemental oxygen until mechanical ventilation is needed (Roussos and Macklem, 1982).

Neurogenic pulmonary oedema is one example of gas exchange failure due to neurological disease. Other examples include pneumonia and pulmonary emboli, both of which are common complications of serious neurological diseases. Most cases of respiratory failure of neurological origin, however, result from failure of adequate pump function.

The ventilatory pump includes the ventilatory muscles, their neural supply, the chest wall, the airways, and the muscles and nerves responsible for upper airway patency. For most people, respiration proceeds automatically, requiring no conscious control and responding to the changing needs of the organism without perceptible effort. Thus, most of the central nervous system components that control respiration are subcortical and are concentrated in the lower brainstem.

No single brainstem centre for respiration exists; instead a collection of diffuse groups of neurones located in areas of the pons and medulla interact to provide automatic control of respiration. Within the medulla, two cell populations have been defined: an inspiratory nucleus, which when stimulated induces sustained inspiration; and an expiratory nucleus, which induces forced expiration. A third group of cells, comprising the pneumotaxic centre of the pons, interacts with the medullary centres to coordinate breathing. At the pontomedullary junction there is a chemoreceptor region which provides information concerning the cerebrospinal fluid concentration of carbon dioxide.

Although respiration continues in the deafferented brainstem, inputs to the brainstem centres are necessary for normal homeostatic control of respiration. Descending inputs have been identified from the cerebral hemispheres, the hypothalamus, and the rostral part of the brainstem. Stimulation experiments have demonstrated the effects of cerebral influences on respiration. For example, stimulation of certain deep frontal and temporal lobe structures induces apnoea, and pyriform cortex stimulation results in tachypnoea.

Peripheral afferents to respiratory centres include vagal and

151

glossopharyngeal inputs from several sources: peripheral chemo-receptors, the carotid sinuses, the aortic arch, the tracheobronchial tree, and mechanoreceptors of respiratory muscles and lungs. These afferents provide a wide variety of information to the brainstem respiratory centres. Peripheral baroreceptors provide information concerning systematic blood pressure; when blood pressure rises, respiratory drive is depressed. Peripheral chemoreceptors allow respiration to respond to changing blood concentrations of oxygen, carbon dioxide, and acid. Sensory inputs from the trachea and bronchi participate in cough reflexes. Transection of the vagus nerves results in slower, deeper respiration with inspiratory and expiratory pauses.

The brainstem respiratory centres integrate information from central and peripheral afferents. Outflow from these centres traverses the lower brainstem to lower motor neurones of the medulla and cervical and thoracic spinal cord. Other upper motor neurones allow voluntary control of respiration; these neurones originate in the cortex and pass in the lateral corticospinal tract. From the lower motor neurone cells of origin in the anterior horn the peripheral nerves exit via cranial nerves IX, X and XI, and cervical and thoracic roots. These peripheral nerves include the left and right phrenic nerves, which innervate the diaphragm, the anterior thoracic nerves, and the intercostal nerves. The diaphragm is the most important muscle of inspiration, but accessory muscles contribute, including the intercostals, scalenes, pectorals, and ster-nocleidomastoids, particularly during forced inspiration. Expiration is facilitated by elastic recoil of the lungs and chest wall, but during forced expiration the abdominal muscles and internal intercostals are active.

## Sites of impairment

Respiratory dysfunction may result from abnormalities involving any portion of the neural and muscular elements of the respiratory system. In some cases, these abnormalities may be relatively mild and may not induce significant respiratory embarrassment; in others, acute respiratory failure may develop within minutes.

Lesions of the cortex and basal ganglia may produce disordered breathing including excessively slow or fast respiration, breath holding, prolonged sighs, inversion of the inspiration/expiration ratio (normally about 1:2), excessive yawning, and spasmodic coughs or hiccups, but they rarely result in frank respiratory failure. Dystonic reactions which involve the upper airway are exceptions; some cases of sudden death in patients receiving phenothiazines may have been due to dystonia of laryngeal and pharyngeal muscles resulting in airway obstruction (Flaherty and Lahmeyer, 1978; Solomon, 1977). Tetanus, another exception, can produce severe respiratory compromise by inducing spasm of respiratory muscles (Davis et al., 1980). In contrast, the hypoventilation or apnoea that commonly occurs during and immediately after generalised tonic–clonic seizures rarely results in life-threatening respiratory failure. Apart from these few exceptions, cerebral lesions do not induce respiratory failure until brainstem function is affected.

Since control of respiration is vested in the brainstem, brainstem lesions are important causes of respiratory failure. Brainstem infarctions or haemorrhages, tumours of the posterior fossa, and hydrocephalus can all result in respiratory failure. Overdoses of sedative, hypnotic and narcotic drugs cause respiratory failure by depressing the activity of the brainstem respiratory centres.

Tumours of the cervico-medullary junction and spinal injuries above the mid-cervical level can be associated with severe respiratory compromise, but when spinal cord injuries occur below the mid-cervical level, the cervical origin of the phrenic nerves spares the diaphragm from paralysis even when other respiratory muscles are affected. However, the paralysis of the abdominal muscles which results from any level of cervical or thoracic spine injury impairs the rapid development of expiratory airway pressure that is necessary for an effective cough.

Anterior horn cell diseases produce respiratory failure when the nerves to the respiratory and upper airway are affected. Although paralytic poliomyelitis is now rarely seen in Western countries, it remains an important cause of acute respiratory failure in areas in which the disease is still endemic. Bulbar poliomyelitis can produce respiratory failure due to pulmonary aspiration, and cervical and thoracic anterior horn cell involvement produces paralysis of the chest wall and diaphragm. Amytrophic lateral sclerosis is frequently associated with respiratory failure for similar reasons.

Lesions affecting several cervical and thoracic nerves and nerve roots can also produce respiratory failure. These lesions occur in Guillain-Barré syndrome as well as in the less common diphtheritic polyneuropathy.

Adequate function of the neuromuscular junction is critical for respiration. Failure of neuromuscular transmission can lead to respiratory impairment and frank respiratory failure in myasthenia gravis, botulism and tick paralysis.

Primary muscle diseases typically cause unequal but symmetric involvement of muscle groups (Aldrich and Aldrich, 1986). When the muscles of respiration are affected, respiratory failure may occur. Although the most severe respiratory involvement of any of the muscular dystrophies occurs with Duchenne muscular dystrophy, diaphragm involvement may be substantial in acid maltase deficiency and limb girdle dystrophy, and respiratory impairment is common in patients with myotonic dystrophy and polymyositis.

## Mechanisms of pump failure

There are four major consequences of abnormal function of the neuromuscular elements of the respiratory system: muscular weakness, neuromuscular fatigue, upper airway obstruction, and impaired coordination of respiratory muscles.

Muscle weakness can result from decreased functional muscle mass, from impaired muscle contractile mechanisms, or from impaired transmission of neural impulses. When the inspiratory muscles are affected, their decreased ability to generate an intrathoracic vacuum decreases the vital capacity, constituting a restrictive defect of pulmonary function. Expiratory muscle weakness results in an ineffective cough. When diaphragmatic weakness occurs in isolation, orthopnoea may result from marked restriction of thoracic volume by the abdominal contents in the supine position.

Neuromuscular fatigue is an important and often overlooked contributor to respiratory failure. Although there is a range of susceptibility to fatigue among skeletal muscles, any muscle can be fatigued if it is subjected to a severe enough load. Fatigue is usually resolved promptly by rest, although some types of fatigue may last more than 24 hours in spite of rest (Edwards, 1979). Increased susceptibility to fatigue can result from any condition, including the effects of inadequate exercise or immobility, which decreases the endurance of a muscle relative to the workload to which it is subjected. In neuromuscular diseases, both respiratory muscle weakness and increased respiratory workload are often present.

For the respiratory muscles, high endurance rather than static strength is required, so fatigue of myopathic respiratory muscles may be even more important than their weakness in causing symptoms. Unusually high susceptibility to fatigue is a hallmark of myasthenia gravis and is characteristic of some of the mitochondrial myopathies.

Upper airway obstruction due to weakness and fatigue of the laryngeal and pharyngeal muscles can result in increased respiratory workload, especially during sleep. During normal inspiratory efforts, contractions of the upper airway muscles oppose the airway narrowing that would otherwise result from the vacuum generated in the thorax. When the upper airway muscles are weakened by bulbar or generalised neuromuscular diseases, partial or complete airway obstruction may occur during inspiration (Aldrich and Sherman, 1985).

Impaired coordination of upper airway or respiratory muscles and impaired muscle relaxation can also produce respiratory dysfunction. Respiratory distress can occur with dystonic reactions from phenothiazines, with respiratory dyskinesias in patients with Parkinson's disease or tardive dyskinesia, and with irregular respirations in patients with Shy–Drager syndrome (Weiner and Klawans, 1980). Impaired relaxation of the respiratory muscles is a special problem for patients with myotonic dystrophy and tetanus, and, occasionally, in Isaac's syndrome.

Respiratory insufficiency may be a problem for some patients only during sleep. Several pathophysiological mechanisms combine to cause nocturnal hypoventilation in some patients who are able to maintain waking ventilation. First, minute ventilation decreases at the onset of sleep. Secondly, tracheal and bronchial stimulation which induces a cough during wakefulness may result in apnoea during sleep. Thirdly, the activity of the accessory muscles of respiration is inhibited during rapid eye movement (REM) sleep, requiring the diaphragm to perform almost all of the work of breathing. Finally, during sleep, postural factors, decreased cortical influences, and diminished tone in airway muscles may precipitate airway closure in patients with otherwise normal airway muscle strength, resulting in the obstructive sleep apnoea syndrome.

Other complications of chronic neuromuscular diseases which affect respiration include kyphoscoliosis, pulmonary emboli, atelectasis, and, most importantly, aspiration pneumonia. Kyphoscoliosis, resulting from the loss of muscular support of the spine, is a frequent complication of Duchenne muscular dystrophy and occasionally complicates other myopathies. The consequent decreased thoracic cage volume and the associated ankylosis of costovertebral joints decrease lung volume and stiffen the chest wall, resulting in large increases in the work of breathing, which, when combined with respiratory muscle weakness, may cause respiratory failure.

Thrombophlebitis and pulmonary embolisation are constant threats to bedridden patients with neurological and neuromuscular diseases. Microatelectasis, which is caused by the rapid shallow breathing without effective sighing, is characteristic of patients with respiratory muscle weakness and results in more lung volume restriction than would be expected from muscle weakness alone. The consequent decreased lung compliance increases the work of breathing.

The combination of aspiration, atelectasis, airway dysfunction, impaired cough and poor clearance of secretions leads to a greatly increased risk of pneumonia in patients with impaired respiratory muscle function. This sequence is frequently the terminal event in these patients.

The remainder of the chapter will be devoted to a discussion of the symptoms and signs of respiratory failure, the approach to diagnosis in these patients, and methods of treatment and prevention of these often fatal complications of neurological diseases.

## SYMPTOMS OF RESPIRATORY FAILURE

Acute respiratory failure may develop either from central causes, in the setting of a catastrophic intracerebral event such as a stroke or haemorrhage, or from peripheral causes, such as a myasthenic crisis or Guillain-Barré syndrome. More often, respiratory failure develops insidiously from progressive weakness due to neuromuscular causes, but only becomes manifest when pneumonia results in decompensation of a patient with marginally compensated respiratory insufficiency. A patient with chronic but manageable respiratory problems may develop acute respiratory failure during a relatively minor viral infection or bronchitis. In each of these cases, swift and accurate diagnosis is essential. The rapidity with which respiratory failure can develop and the devastating consequences of inadequate treatment require the physician to be alert to the possibility of respiratory failure in patients with a wide variety of neurological illnesses.

Patients with known neurological diseases often develop acute respiratory failure, with or without previous respiratory symptoms. A patient with myasthenia gravis, for example, may become relatively refractory to medications following a fever or infectious illness, and may then develop acute respiratory failure . Guillain-Barré syndrome, particularly in the first few days following onset of illness, may progress with such remarkable speed that a patient with no respiratory symptoms will require a ventilator within a few hours of his first neurological symptom. Less commonly, respiratory failure may be the presenting symptom of an otherwise undiagnosed neurological condition such as amyotrophic lateral sclerosis or acid maltase deficiency.

The cardinal symptom of respiratory failure is dyspnoea. Dyspnoea occurring at rest is particularly serious and suggests that the need for assisted ventilation may be imminent. In patients with marginal respiratory function, dyspnoea may not be present at rest but may develop with minimal amounts of exercise such as walking a few steps. When the diaphragm is impaired out of proportion to other muscles of respiration, dyspnoea may be apparent only in the supine position.

When respiratory function is worse during sleep, patients may complain principally of sleep disturbance, including frequent awakenings and nocturnal dyspnoea. On the other hand, the nocturnal sleep disturbance of obstructive sleep apnoea may be unnoticed by the patient, who instead complains of daytime sleepiness or morning headaches. Most of these patients are unaware of the nightly apnoeas; it is their spouses who bring them to the attention of the physician.

## SIGNS ASSOCIATED WITH RESPIRATORY FAILURE

The physical signs that are associated with respiratory failure depend on its cause. The causes can be divided into those that affect the central respiratory centres and those that affect the pathways from these centres to the respiratory muscles.

### Signs associated with central causes of respiratory failure

Patients with brain and brainstem causes of abnormal respiration show characteristic changes of breathing pattern which are useful in determining the affected areas of the central nervous system (Table 9.1). Since these patients are usually stuporous or comatose and unable to complain of respiratory distress, it is particularly important to recognise the signs which indicate impending respiratory failure.

**Table 9.1:** Typical breathing patterns associated with brain injury

| Area of brain injury | Breathing pattern | Description of breathing |
|---|---|---|
| Bilateral hemispheric lesions | Cheyne-Stokes respiration | Cyclical variation in depth of respiration. Tidal volume increases and decreases smoothly. After a brief period of apnoea the cycle is repeated |
| Midbrain | Sustained hyperpnoea | Rapid, regular, large ventilations of 24–38 per minute |
| Pons | Apneustic breathing | Pause at full inspiration, abnormally prolonged expiration, and an expiratory pause lasting 2–3 seconds |
| Medulla | Ataxic breathing | Irregular respirations without fixed rate or rhythm |

In patients with expanding mass lesions of the brain, such as hemispheric tumours, abscesses, haemorrhages or oedema from head injuries, two characteristic patterns of rostral to caudal deterioration may occur. These are the 'uncal syndrome' and the 'central syndrome' (Plum and Posner, 1980). The two patterns show distinct differences during their early phases, but as the level of dysfunction progresses to the midbrain and below, the differences disappear.

In the uncal syndrome, the most striking clinical feature is the gradually dilating pupil on the same side as the expanding mass, due to compression of the third nerve by the herniating uncus. During this stage of the uncal syndrome, Cheyne-Stokes respirations may be seen. Cheyne-Stokes respirations, a normal phenomenon during infant sleep, can also be seen in patients with uraemia, congestive heart failure or other conditions that produce a prolonged circulation time. In patients with neurological disease, Cheyne-Stokes respirations are most likely to occur in patients with deep bilateral lesions, involving the basal ganglia or internal capsules. Stroke and hypertensive encephalopathy are frequent causes. In the awake or stuporous patient with an expanding supratentorial mass lesion, the Cheyne-Stokes pattern is a sign of neurological dysfunction that should alert the clinician to the possibility of impending transtentorial herniation. However, the Cheyne-Stokes pattern may not occur, and respiration may be entirely normal; consequently, a normal respiratory pattern does not ensure that the patient is clinically stable.

As the uncal syndrome progresses, midbrain dysfunction rapidly develops with coma and ophthalmoplegia. Cheyne-Stokes respirations or central neurogenic hyperventilation may occur. With further progression, the changes in the respiratory pattern are the same as those occurring with the central syndrome described below. Not infrequently, the central and uncal syndromes occur together, and the development of a third-nerve palsy is associated with Cheyne-Stokes respiration and stupor.

The first or diencephalic stage of the central syndrome is characterised clinically by a change in the level of alertness. The patient may be agitated, confused, drowsy or stuporous. The pupils are typically small and the eye movements may be conjugate or may be roving and slightly divergent. Hemiparesis or hemiplegia may be present. Repeated sighs and yawns may occur, and Cheyne-Stokes respirations may be present.

As brainstem dysfunction progresses, midbrain impairment is indicated clinically by coma with decerebrate or decorticate rigidity, and by fixed, midposition pupils of moderate size. The pattern of Cheyne-Stokes respiration typically gives way gradually to sustained hyperpnoea, often described as central neurogenic hyperventilation. Although central neurogenic hyperventilation is associated with a worse prognosis than Cheyne-Stokes respiration, recovery can still occur.

The cause of the hyperpnoea associated with midbrain lesions is controversial. Although the term 'central neurogenic hyperventilation' implies a primary neurological cause, animal studies have failed to produce a similar syndrome. Most patients with a diagnosis of central neurogenic hyperventilation have been found to have pulmonary congestion at autopsy. More recently, it has been suggested that pulmonary congestion produces hyperventilation as a result of increased activity of peripheral afferents arising in the lung and chest wall (Plum and Posner, 1980). Most patients with hyperpnoea in the setting of coma from brainstem dysfunction have respiratory alkalosis and an arterial $PO_2$ below that expected for the degree of hypocapnia, suggesting the presence of pulmonary dysfunction such as shunting. The weight of evidence therefore indicates that in most cases central neurogenic hyperventilation is caused by neurogenic pulmonary oedema.

When the level of brainstem dysfunction progresses to the lower pons, the tidal volume decreases, although a rapid and more or less regular pattern of respiration may continue. Eye movements cease, even with caloric stimulation, and the patient becomes flaccid.

As the level of dysfunction continues to progress to the upper medulla, the pathways connecting respiratory centres are disrupted, the respiratory rate declines, and ataxic respirations are observed. Ataxic breathing may proceed quickly to respiratory cessation and is especially susceptible to the respiratory depressant effects of sedatives and hypnotics. With continued caudal progression, the rate of respiration slows and long periods of apnoea may occur before breathing finally stops. The blood pressure falls, and the heart rate becomes irregular.

Ataxic breathing may also occur in primary diseases of the posterior fossa. Patients who have developed ataxic breathing from rostral–caudal deterioration have a poor prognosis, but when posterior fossa lesions are the cause the prognosis is less certain and many patients will recover following surgical decompression. Ataxic breathing may be caused by cerebellar haemorrhage and infarction, and by medullary infarction from bilateral vertebral artery occlusion. Acute para-infectious brainstem demyelination from poliovirus or other viral infections is another cause of ataxic breathing.

Apneustic breathing is most commonly caused by infarction affecting the pneumotaxic centre in the lower pons, but may also be seen in association with anoxic brain injury, meningitis, or coma from hypoglycaemia. Although apneustic breathing seldom if ever occurs with herniation syndromes, it may alternate with other centrally mediated abnormal breathing patterns.

Another rare cause of respiratory failure is failure of automatic breathing while asleep. In this condition, respiration is normal or nearly normal during wakefulness, but severe hypoventilation is present during sleep. This entity has been called 'Ondine's curse',[1] or central alveolar hypoventilation, and may occur in association with diseases of the medulla which damage the respiratory centres but leave intact the corticospinal pathways to respiratory motor neurones. Consequently, voluntary respiration can be carried out, but automatic respiration is impaired. These patients generally do not complain of dyspnoea.

Neurogenic pulmonary oedema is an important cause of respiratory failure in patients with acute intracranial processes. Although the incidence of neurogenic pulmonary oedema has not been established, it appears to be a frequent cause acute respiratory failure in patients with intracranial catastrophes due to head injury, intracranial haemorrhage, seizures, and brain tumours. Neurogenic pulmonary oedema has been reproduced in experimental animals following head injury; in these animals, pulmonary oedema develops within seconds or minutes after head injury. The pathophysiological basis appears to be leakage of fluid into the interstitial lung space, due to increased capillary permeability at a time of greatly increased systemic blood pressure and associated increased pulmonary blood volume (Hoff et al., 1981). The cause of the sudden increase in blood pressure, called 'vasomotor storm', is not known. The possibility of neurogenic pulmonary oedema should be considered in any patient with an acute central nervous system catastrophe who develops signs of respiratory insufficiency.

By the time neurogenic pulmonary oedema becomes clinically apparent, the blood pressure has usually returned to normal. The initial clinical features are dyspnoea, tachypnoea, and tachycardia. End-expiratory crackles are heard on chest auscultation. In severe cases, clear or pink-tinged frothy sputum may be evident. The chest radiograph usually shows a diffuse fluffy pattern of alveolar infiltrates, the 'bat-wing' appearance, although unilateral infiltrates are occasionally seen. Arterial blood gases initially show respiratory alkalosis with hypoxaemia but, as the clinical picture worsens, respiratory acidosis and hypercarbia may supervene.

In mild cases, it may be possible to oxygenate the patient adequately with supplemental oxygen delivered via a nasal cannula or face mask; more commonly, endotracheal intubation and assisted ventilation are required. In severe cases, positive end-expiratory pressure (PEEP) is required. Increased intracranial pressure, if present, should be controlled with osmotic diuretics, hyperventilation, and/or corticosteroids, since marked or prolonged increased intracranial pressure probably contributes to or worsens neurogenic pulmonary oedema, and the use of mechanical ventilation and PEEP may aggravate the intracranial hypertension. Neurogenic pulmonary oedema may resolve within hours or it may persist for several days, depending somewhat on the severity of the neurological problem.

## Signs associated with peripheral causes of respiratory failure

Tachypnoea is the most sensitive sign in patients with peripheral causes of respiratory impairment. The respirations of patients with restrictive ventilatory defects due to respiratory muscle weakness are usually rapid and shallow. If the weakness of the diaphragm is out of proportion to that of other respiratory muscles, the action of accessory muscles is proportionately increased and the consequent cephalad motion of the weakened diaphragm during inspiration will then cause paradoxical inward abdominal movements, the so-called 'abdominal paradox'. Conversely, if intercostal and accessory muscles are paralysed, the action of the diaphragm alone may produce inward movements of the thorax during inspiration. Weakness of expiratory muscles is not apparent during normal breathing movements; however, a weak cough often indicates weakness of the expiratory muscles.

End-inspiratory crackles on chest auscultation may be caused by microatelectasis from incomplete inspiration and inadequate sighing. Alternatively, they may accompany interstitial pulmonary oedema from neurogenic cardiogenic causes. Early inspiratory crackles may be the result of inadequate clearance of secretions. Kyphoscoliosis sufficiently severe also to impair pulmonary function is readily detectable on physical examination and implies long-standing weakness of spinal musculature. Cyanosis may be present and lethargy may reflect the effects of hypoxia or hypercapnia. True excessive sleepiness suggests impaired pulmonary function during sleep, and is a prominent symptom when obstructive sleep apnoea is present and when sleep apnoea complicates marginal daytime respiratory function.

In patients with neuromuscular causes of respiratory failure, associated neurological signs are almost always present. Patients with myopathies usually have proximal muscle weakness, with involvement of neck flexors. Patients with myasthenia gravis usually have impaired ocular and bulbar muscle function, and fatiguable weakness of proximal muscles can sometimes be demonstrated with repetitive strength testing of the deltoids, neck flexors, and other proximal muscles. In some patients with laryngeal and pharyngeal weakness, dysarthria is apparent during routine speech; in others, repetition of phrases such as 'Coca-Cola, Coca-Cola. . .' may demonstrate weakness or easy fatiguability of the palatal muscles. Impaired ability to swallow can be tested easily at the bedside, with care to avoid aspiration. Muscles innervated by cervical roots can be tested in patients with Guillain-Barré syndrome and other diseases of nerves and nerve roots. Motor neurone disease severe enough to produce respiratory failure is almost always associated with atrophy and fasciculations of the muscles of the chest wall or arms.

## DIAGNOSTIC EVALUATION

Accurate diagnosis of both the neurological and the respiratory components is essential for the management of the patient with respiratory failure of neurological origin. In most cases of central origin, the associated neurological findings of coma, hemiparesis, ataxia, or oculomotor or pupillary abnormalities will help to locate the neurological lesion, and computed tomography can determine whether intracranial haemorrhage has occurred. In cases of peripheral origin, the presence or absence of sensory abnormalities, reflex changes, tongue and chest wall fasciculations, and the results of nerve conduction studies and electromyography can help to determine the site of the abnormality and its pathogenesis. With regard to the respiratory component, five types of investigation can be used to determine the cause and to asses the course of either failure of gas exchange or failure of pump function. These investigations are: the physical examination, the chest roentgenogram, pulmonary function tests, the arterial blood gas measurements, and the sputum examination.

### Physical examination

The respiratory rate and pattern can be helpful in identifying the site of an intracranial lesion as outlined earlier. In addition, tachypnoea serves as a non-specific indication of respiratory function impairment, since it occurs in patients with respiratory muscle weakness or fatigue, atelectasis, chest wall restriction, pneumonia and pulmonary embolism. Supraclavicular retractions and visible contractions of sternomastoid or intercostal muscles usually indicate excessive respiratory workload, with impaired respiratory reserve. Inspiratory inward motion of the abdomen suggests marked diaphragmatic weakness or fatigue. The presence of pneumonia, pleural effusion, or lobar atelectasis is usually readily detectable on physical examination.

### Chest Roentgenogram

The chest roentgenogram is an essential part of the evaluation of any patient with respiratory failure of neurological origin. Bilateral interstitial and alveolar infiltrates are characteristic of neurogenic

163

pulmonary oedema. Regional hypovascularity or a peripheral wedge-shaped infiltrate may signify pulmonary embolism. Basilar atelectasis and pneumonic infiltrates are readily detectable. In combination with fluoroscopy, paradoxical diaphragmatic movement can be detected.

## Pulmonary function tests

The vital capacity, the maximum volume of air that can be exhaled or inhaled in one continuous breath, is the single most useful test of overall respiratory function, especially for patients with non-central impairments. The vital capacity is reduced with respiratory muscle weakness and by such mechanical impairments as airway obstruction, stiff lungs, or chest wall restriction. A simple hand-held spirometer (for example, the Mechanical Spirometer Model 8800, Boehringer Laboratories, Inc., Wynnewood, PA, USA) can be used to determine the vital capacity with acceptable accuracy; its only drawback is the inability of some patients to perform the manoeuvre on command or to create a tight seal over the mouthpiece.

Another useful pair of bedside tests of respiratory function is the maximal inspiratory airway pressure ($PI_{max}$) and the maximal expiratory airway pressure ($PE_{max}$) (Black and Hyatt, 1971). $PI_{max}$ is the maximal negative airway pressure that can be generated during momentary airway occlusion at functional residual capacity (the resting end-expiratory lung volume). $PE_{max}$ is the maximal positive airway pressure during airway occlusion at total lung capacity. Because they are measured during a period of absent airflow, the mouth pressure changes are identical to the intrathoracic pressure changes and thus accurately reflect either the inspiratory ($PI_{max}$) or expiratory ($PE_{max}$) muscle strength (Figure 9.2). Respiratory muscle weakness can often be differentiated from abnormal pulmonary mechanics by comparison of the degree of impairment in the maximal mouth pressures with that of the vital capacity.

In some cases, especially when there is coexistent primary pulmonary disease, or when bedside tests are not adequate for an accurate diagnosis, more complete pulmonary testing is helpful. Such tests generally include spirometry, during which the forced expiratory volume in one second (FEV-1) and the ratio of the FEV-1 to the vital capacity serve as indices of airway obstruction. The results of spirometry, typically displayed as a flow-volume loop, can confirm the presence of a restrictive defect in pulmonary function,

**Figure 9.2:** Apparatus used to measure vital capacity and maximal inspiratory and expiratory mouth pressures in seriously ill patients. For patients with cuffed endotracheal or tracheostomy tubes, the T-piece can be connected directly. For patients breathing through the mouth, a mouthpiece is used, and the nose is clipped. For the vital capacity measurement, the patient is asked to breathe in as deeply as possible, then to blow out as much air as possible. The exhaled air is measured using the spirometer (these instruments are designed for relatively low flow rates; high flow rates can damage them). For the peak inspiratory pressure measurement, the inspiratory valve is occluded with the stopper after a full expiration (functional residual capacity) and the patient is asked to make a maximal inspiratory effort. Several sequential efforts may be required before the true maximal negative pressure is attained. The small leak created by the 14-gauge needle is needed when efforts are made via a mouthpiece, in order to prevent spurious results due to suction with the palatal muscles. For measurements of $PE_{max}$, the stopper is used on the expiratory valve and the measurement is started from total lung capacity

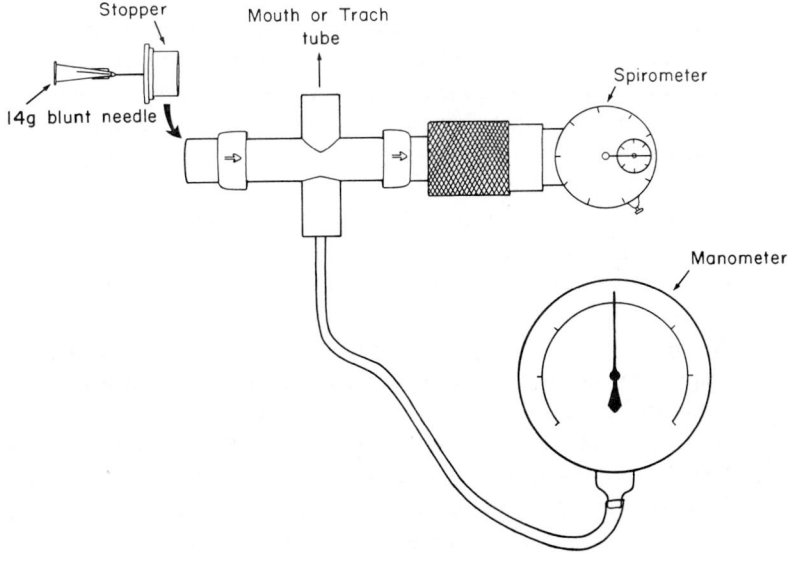

but they cannot reliably differentiate pulmonary from respiratory muscle causes of such restriction.

## Tests of diaphragm function

The diaphragm is the most important respiratory muscle. The strength of the diaphragm can be assessed with reasonable accuracy by determination of the maximal transdiaphragmatic pressure using oesophageal and gastric balloon catheters. Fluoroscopy of the diaphragm is useful for the detection of diaphragmatic paralysis, which is manifested by 'paradoxical' cephalad displacement of one or both hemidiaphragms during an inspiratory effort. Diaphragmatic fluoroscopy should be performed in the supine and upright position, and abdominal muscle activity should be monitored to avoid misinterpretation of results due to abdominal muscle contraction. Diaphragm electromyography (EMG) and phrenic nerve stimulation studies may be helpful if diaphragmatic denervation or fatigue is suspected.

## Arterial blood gases

Arterial blood gases can detect life-threatening hypoxaemia or impending ventilatory failure, as manifested by hypercapnia and respiratory acidosis. Blood gases are not, however, a sensitive measure of respiratory impairment, since they may remain normal at rest even when marked respiratory muscle weakness is present. In fact, resting hypercapnia develops only when the respiratory muscle strength falls below about 50% of predicted (Braun et al., 1983). In many patients with respiratory muscle weakness of peripheral origin, especially when diaphragmatic weakness is prominent, hypercapnia and hypoxaemia become much worse during sleep. Primary metabolic acidosis with compensatory respiratory alkalosis in a comatose patient with tachypnoea suggests a metabolic cause of coma such as hyperglycaemia or uraemia. Arterial blood gases will help to differentiate these conditions from hepatic encephalopathy, which may have an associated respiratory alkalosis, and from pulmonary oedema or pneumonia, which are often associated with respiratory alkalosis.

## Sputum examination

Sputum examination is simple, inexpensive, and invaluable when bronchitis or pneumonia is suspected. The appearance of sputum can provide clues about the severity of the infection. In many cases, the pathogenic organism can be promptly identified by microscopic examination of stained specimens. If sputum samples cannot be obtained because the patient is unable to cough, nasotracheal aspiration may be helpful.

## Specialised testing

Ventilation and perfusion scintiscans are particularly helpful in the patient with suspected pulmonary embolism. Areas of decreased uptake of radionuclide on perfusion scan may be due to pulmonary emboli or they may be due to diminished perfusion of poorly ventilated lung regions, pneumonia, atelectasis, or airway obstruction. However, when combined with evidence of adequate ventilation by physical examination, chest roentgenogram, and, preferably, xenon ventilation scan, the diagnosis of pulmonary embolism is relatively secure.

Tests of carbon dioxide responsiveness are helpful in assessing central abnormalities of respiratory drive. Normally, with carbon dioxide inhalation, ventilation and airway occlusion pressure (a measure of respiratory drive) increase. Smaller than normal increases in ventilation or occlusion pressure suggest the presence of impaired respiratory drive.

Polysomnography can provide useful information in patients with suspected sleep apnoea, or in patients with borderline daytime respiratory function who develop sleep disturbances. The sleep study should include monitoring of blood oxygen by ear oximeter, as well as electroencephalogram, chin EMG, and eye movements to permit sleep stage identification. Simultaneous monitoring of airflow and respiratory effort will help distinguish obstructive from non-obstructive apnoea. Periods of decreased respiratory effort with hypoxaemia may occur during REM sleep due to weakness of the diaphragm.

## PREVENTION AND TREATMENT

For many patients who are nearly or totally immobilised by neurological illness, prevention of respiratory complications can mean the difference between death and a return to normal function. Patients with Guillain-Barré syndrome, myasthenia gravis, head

167

injuries, strokes and spinal cord trauma may require many months of rehabilitation. During this time, they are especially vulnerable to respiratory complications, including pulmonary embolisation and aspiration pneumonia.

Prevention and treatment of respiratory failure must be directed at the underlying neurological and respiratory causes. In addition to specific measures directed at the disease processes, a number of general guidelines are applicable in most of these patients. For example, in patients with chronic neuromuscular diseases, obesity and cigarette smoking may aggravate respiratory symptoms and should be eliminated.

Adequate nutrition is often overlooked in patients with respiratory failure. Malnutrition weakens the respiratory muscles, often to a severe degree (Arora and Rochester, 1982). On the other hand, nutritional support, especially with large amounts of carbohydrates, can increase carbon dioxide production, leading to increased ventilatory requirements and consequent increased work of breathing (Covelli *et al.*, 1981). In general, the beneficial effects of prevention of respiratory muscle atrophy outweigh the deleterious effects.

The approach to the prevention of pulmonary embolisation depends on the clinical setting. Most ambulatory patients are at little risk and require no therapy; thus a patient with respiratory failure due to amyotrophic lateral sclerosis who retains significant strength in the extremities should be encouraged to continue to walk or move about. For patients with acute respiratory failure who are largely immobilised, such as a patient in coma or one with Guillain-Barré syndrome, a low dose of heparin (5000 units subcutaneously every 12 hours) is recommended. For patients with established venous thrombosis or previous pulmonary embolisation, full-dose anticoagulation is recommended for at least 6 months or until the risk factors are controlled. Intravenous heparin at a dose sufficient to attain a partial thromboplastin time of greater than 60 seconds is necessary until an appropriate oral dose of warfarin can be determined. For bed-bound paralysed patients, lifetime therapy is indicated.

Prevention of pneumonia is an equally vital aim of medical and nursing care in patients who are immobilised by neurological illnesses. The rapid shallow breathing observed in patients with poor respiratory muscle strength may cause microatelectasis, which in turn provides an ideal setting for proliferation of microorganisms and consequent pneumonia. Microatelectasis can usually be avoided if such patients are capable of an occasional deep sigh; the incentive spirometer is a useful device for encouraging frequent sighing in patients with enough residual muscle strength. In comatose patients with tracheostomies, frequent large-volume assisted breaths by Ambu bag accomplish the same purpose.

Lobar atelectasis is an occasional complication of neuromuscular diseases, occurring either as a result of the same mechanisms that promote microatelectasis, or as a result of bronchial occlusion by an aspirated foreign body. The consequent decreased local clearance of mucus may further obstruct the airway. Postural drainage and suction can usually clear the obstruction sufficiently to allow reinflation, but fibreoptic bronchoscopy may occasionally be necessary to remove a foreign body or a particularly tenacious plug.

Recurrent aspiration is a major threat for patients with neuromuscular diseases. Preventive measures include elevation of the head of the bed to 15°, avoidance of meals within an hour of bedtime, and the use of antacids at bedtime. Swallowing with the head forward, and coughing after each bite, will help to minimise aspiration in patients with neuromuscular diseases. For these patients, liquids may be easier to swallow than solid food. In comatose patients and in those with severe muscle weakness and dysphagia, periodic suctioning of the mouth and pharynx may be helpful.

Neither endotracheal intubation not tracheostomy prevents aspiration, even when cuffed tubes are used. Nasogastric feeding bypasses the pharynx, but since the presence of the nasogastric tube compromises the security of the gastro-oesophageal junction and promotes regurgitation of gastric contents into the mouth, it may be counterproductive. When tube feedings are necessary, soft, weighted duodenal tubes of small calibre, which deposit the feedings distal to the pyloric valve, are preferable to large nasogastric tubes. Gastrostomy or jejunostomy occasionally becomes necessary when repeated aspirations threaten seriously to impair pulmonary function.

The infectious complications of aspiration can be recognised by sputum examinations. The usual pathogens are gram-negative or anaerobic organisms, and the antibiotic regimen should be tailored accordingly. Patients with superimposed reversible airways disease benefit from the use of bronchodilators. The acute deterioration in pulmonary function is usually reversible, and, when the immediate problem is resolved, pulmonary function will usually return to the level that existed prior to the pneumonia.

169

Aminophylline is useful for the treatment of bronchospasm. Recent evidence has suggested that aminophylline and other methylxanthines may also improve the endurance of normal respiratory and other muscles (Aubier *et al.*, 1981), but it is still uncertain whether the endurance of myopathic muscles can be improved with aminophylline. Benzodiazepines, barbiturates and antispastic agents should be avoided in most patients with neuromuscular diseases, because these drugs reduce respiratory drive. Aminoglycoside antibiotics may enhance neuromuscular blockade and should also be avoided if possible. In an occasional patient, a respiratory stimulant such as doxepram, protriptyline, or medroxyprogesterone acetate may improve respiratory drive.

In comatose patients, rapid control of increased intracranial pressure is mandatory. When there is evidence of increased pressure, endotracheal intubation and mechanical hyperventilation are necessary. The partial pressure of carbon dioxide ($PCO_2$) should be lowered to 25 torr: typical volume-cycled ventilator settings to achieve this level of $PCO_2$ are a ventilation rate of 24 and a tidal volume of 1200 cm$^3$ (cc). Intravenous mannitol (25–75 g) should be given and repeated as needed to lower intracranial pressure, which can be measured with an intracranial monitor. In patients with brain tumours, high doses of dexamethasone may provide a temporary reduction of intracranial pressure; however, in patients with cytotoxic brain oedema from stroke, steroids are rarely effective.

In patients with respiratory failure of peripheral origin, due to myasthenia gravis or Guillain-Barré syndrome, mechanical ventilation may be required for weeks to months. The decision to initiate intubation and mechanical ventilation should be based on measurements of the patient's vital capacity and negative inspiratory pressure ($PI_{max}$). The rate of decline of the vital capacity is more important than the actual value. It is much better to intubate the patient in a controlled setting with appropriate preparation when the vital capacity falls below 1000 cm$^3$ than it is to wait for acute respiratory failure and carbon dioxide retention. Small doses of intravenous diazepam just before intubation will often induce amnesia for the procedure. Once the patient is intubated, the initial ventilator settings should be such that no voluntary ventilation is required; for example, tidal volume of 10–12 cm$^3$/kg and a rate of 10–14/minute. At these settings. the respiratory muscles can be rested and respiratory muscle fatigue can be relieved. Periodic sighs of 15–20 cm$^3$/kg should be administered in order to prevent atelectasis.

The subsequent course of ventilator management depends on the cause of respiratory failure. In myasthenia gravis, in which a period of complete rest of respiratory muscles is beneficial, anticholinesterase agents are either reduced in dosage or temporarily discontinued; treatment is directed at associated pulmonary infections or other complications. A few days without anticholinesterase agents often results in increased responsiveness to these medications. When the pulmonary status is optimal, anticholinesterase agents are gradually reintroduced or increased to maximise vital capacity and negative inspiratory pressure. Once the pulmonary complications or systemic infections are eliminated, ventilatory weaning is usually not difficult. If anticholinesterase agents alone are insufficient, such ancillary treatments as plasmaphoresis, corticosteroids, and thymectomy may be necessary. These treatments are best undertaken at centres experienced in the management of severe myasthenia gravis.

Patients with Guillain-Barré syndrome who develop respiratory failure usually have a prolonged course; the average length of ventilatory support is 40 days. Volume-cycled ventilators provide better control of minute ventilation than pressure-cycled ventilators; initially, the ventilator is set in the *control* mode so that the patient's entire ventilatory needs are satisfied mechanically. A tidal volume of 10–12 cm$^3$/kg and a rate of 10–14/minute are usually adequate. Fractional inspired oxygen concentration (FiO$_2$) can be determined by the patient's arterial blood gases. Weaning from the ventilator should not be attempted until the patient's vital capacity and negative inspiratory pressure have approached values of 10 cm$^3$/kg and 20 cm H$_2$O respectively. We recommend beginning with brief periods of 10–20 minutes off the ventilator using a T-tube. As respiratory muscle strength increases, these periods are lengthened. Assisted ventilation at night may be required for some time even when daytime waking ventilation is adequate.

In some patients with such chronic irreversible neuromuscular diseases as amyotrophic lateral sclerosis and muscular dystrophy, it may not be possible to discontinue assisted ventilation once it has been initiated. Many of these patients can be successfully treated at home with ventilatory assist devices. It may be possible to limit assisted ventilation to cuirass ventilators (which compress the chest externally and do not require tracheostomy) or positive pressure ventilators used during sleep. For those who require full-time mechanical ventilation, portable respirators are available and can be attached to a wheelchair.

The decision to use assisted ventilation indefinitely is not an easy one. It is best for the patient and his family to become fully acquainted with the various techniques of assisted ventilation and the implications for daily living *before* the need for ventilatory support is imminent. If the patient does decide to use ventilatory assist devices, he should be permitted to choose to discontinue these devices at some later date.

## SUMMARY

Respiratory failure can occur in a wide variety of neurological illnesses; it may develop acutely, or respiratory insufficiency may progress insidiously over a number of months or years. Prompt and accurate diagnosis of both the neurological illness and the respiratory abnormality is necessary for optimal treatment, and is facilitated by accurate interpretation of findings on physical examination and by the use of appropriate laboratory tests. In many instances the neurological disorder causing respiratory failure is reversible, and treatment is directed at maintaining adequate ventilation until the patient improves. Even when the underlying neurological disorder is not treatable, a variety of treatments are available which may alleviate the pulmonary abnormality.

## NOTE

1. According to German legend, Ondine, a water nymph, is jilted by her mortal lover, Hans. In retaliation, she puts a curse on him, such that he must voluntarily remember to breathe. Since his breathing is not automatic, when he finally falls asleep he dies.

## REFERENCES

Aldrich, T.K. and Aldrich,. M.S. (1986) Primary muscle diseases respiratory mechanisms and complications. In S. Kamholtz (ed.), *Respiratory complications of neurologic disease*, SP Medical/Scientific Books, New York

Aldrich, T.K. and Sherman, M.S. (1985) Inspiratory upper airway construction in neuromuscular diseases. *Clin. Res. 33*, 461A

Arora, N.S. and Rochester, D.F. (1982) Respiratory muscle strength and maximal voluntary ventilation in undernourished patients. *Am. Rev. Respir. Dis. 126*, 5–8

Aubier, M., DeTroyer, A., Sampson, M., Macklem, P.T. and Roussos, C. (1981) Aminophylline improves diaphragmatic contractility. *New Engl. J. Med.* 305, 249–52

Black, L.F. and Hyatt, R.E. (1971) Maximal static respiratory pressures in generalised neuromuscular disease. *Am. Rev. Respir. Dis.* 103, 641–50

Braun, N.M.T., Arora, N.S. and Rochester, D.F. (1983) Respiratory muscle and pulmonary function in polymyositis and other proximal myopathies. *Thorax* 38, 616–23

Covelli, H.D., Black, J.W., Olsen, M.S. and Beekman, J. (1981) Respiratory failure precipitated by high carbohydrate loads. *Ann. Intern. Med.* 95, 579–81

Davis, L.E., Jackson, D.L. and Gothe, B. (1980) Neurological infections and respiratory dysfunction. In W.J. Weiner (ed.), *Respiratory dysfunction in neurologic disease*, Futura, New York

Edwards, R.H.T. (1979) The diaphragm as a muscle: mechanisms underlying fatigue. *Am. Rev. Respir. Dis.* 119 (Part 2), 81–4

Flaherty, J.A. and Lahmeyer, H.W. (1978) Laryngeal–pharyngeal dystonia as a possible cause of asphyxia with haloperidol treatment. *Am. J. Psychiat.* 135, 1414–15

Gilroy, J., Cahalan, J.L., Berman, R. and Newman, M. (1963) Cardiac and pulmonary complications in Duchenne's progressive muscular dystrophy. *Circulation* 27, 484–89

Hoff, J.T., Nishimura, M., Garcia-Uria, J. and Miranda, S. (1981) Experimental neurogenic pulmonary edema. *J. Neurosurg.* 54, 627–31

Inkley, S.R., Oldenberg, F.C. and Vignos, P.J. (1974) Pulmonary function in Duchenne's muscular dystrophy related to stage of disease. *Am. J. Med.* 56, 297–306

Plum, F. and Posner, J.B. (1980) *The diagnosis of stupor and coma*, F.A. Davis, Philadelphia

Roussos, C. and Macklem, P.T. (1982) The respiratory muscles. *New Engl. J. Med.* 307, 786–97

Solomon, K. (1977) Phenothiazine-induced bulbar palsy-like syndrome and sudden death. *Am. J. Psychiat.* 134, 308–11

Weiner, W.J. and Klawans, H.L. (1980) Respiratory dysfunction in movement disorders. In W.J. Weiner (ed.) *Respiratory dysfunction in neurologic disease*, Futura, New York

# 10

# Acute Visual Failure

Simon Harding and Peter Sandercock

## INTRODUCTION

In this chapter we will consider the problem of acute visual failure, with a section at the end on acute onset diplopia. Local eye problems may be difficult to distinguish from neurological causes of visual loss, and so we have included a description of primarily ocular diseases. We present the topic not in textbook fashion but rather in a simple logical manner which should allow the non-ophthalmologist to arrive at an accurate diagnosis. We do not have the space to cover treatment in detail except where emergency action is required. We feel that most cases will require referral to a specialist and have indicated as far as possible whether it should be an ophthalmologist or a neurologist.

## HISTORY

The following points should be established in a brief history:

(a) *Onset*. Speed of onset suggests the causative mechanism. Vascular causes are sudden, with arterial occlusions often being described as being 'as though someone switched off the light' or 'a curtain suddenly came down over the eye', and venous occlusions as being 'as though someone dimmed the light before switching it off'.

(b) *Pain*. Severe pain when associated with sudden loss of vision indicates acute closed angle glaucoma or acute anterior uveitis.

(c) *Unilateral or bilateral*. Beware a homonymous hemianopia. For example, a left homonymous hemianopia may be described as 'loss of vision in the left eye'.

(d) *Intermittent or persistent.*

(e) *Blurred vision or double vision.* Many patients confuse 'double vision' with blurred vision; careful questioning may resolve the problem.

(f) *Associated symptoms.* Other neurological symptoms such as limb weakness, dysphasia and cranial nerve palsies may help localise the problem. Floaters are extremely common, but when their onset is followed by loss of vision retinal detachment must be excluded.

(g) *Previous eye disease.* Previously known senile macular degeneration may suddenly and dramatically deteriorate due to disciform change. Previous retinal detachment or optic nerve disease may suggest the cause of the current complaint.

An important pitfall to beware of is a patient with gradual painless unilateral loss of vision who presents with apparent sudden visual loss. They discover it usually after covering the fellow eye and realising that vision in the affected eye is poor. Commonest causes of this apparent sudden loss of vision are a dense uniocular cataract, chronic open angle glaucoma and senile macular degeneration.

**EXAMINATION**

Accurate ophthalmological diagnosis requires relatively inexpensive and simple equipment (Figure 10.1). Specialist equipment is only necessary to pick up milder grades of chronic disease and for follow-up. The following comprises a standard examination.

*Visual acuity (VA)*

Snellen distance chart tested at 6 m. Near reading type if indicated. Use pinhole to neutralise any refractive error.

*Inspection*

Red and painful eyes with acute visual loss are due to acute closed angle glaucoma or acute anterior uveitis, until proved otherwise.

*Pupils*

Method of testing:

(1) Patient fixes on a *distant* object in a dimly lit room.

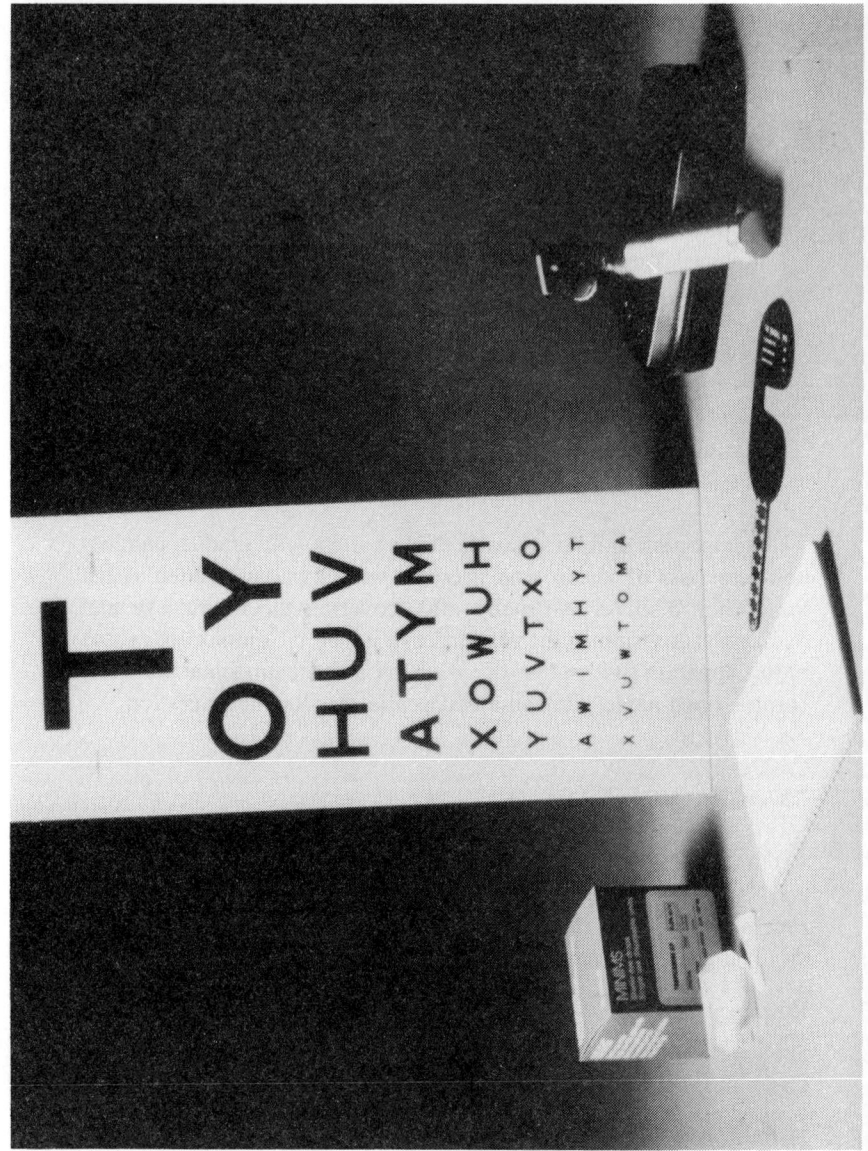

**Figure 10.1:**
Equipment needed for neuro-ophthalmic examination: Snellen chart, ophthalmoscope, near test type, pinhole and tropicamide dilating drops

(2) Shine a *bright* light into one eye and observe
 (a) direct response,
 (b) consensual response.
(3) Shine light into other eye and observe direct and consensual response.
(4) Swinging flashlight test (Figure 10.2). *Rapidly* move the light from one eye to other before pupils have time to dilate. Provided the distance of the light source remains constant, the pupils will *neither dilate nor constrict* because the input to the crossed pupillary pathway is the same whichever eye the light is shone into.
(5) Near response. Only test if a defect is present on light testing. An accommodative target such as lettering is essential; a light source will not induce the near response.

## Common pupillary defects associated with sudden loss of vision

(a) Unilateral fixed and dilated pupil:
 (i) with pain — acute closed angle glaucoma;
 (ii) without pain — suspect pharmacological pupil or third-nerve palsy.
(b) Unilateral fixed and constricted pupil:
 (i) with pain — acute anterior uveitis;
 (ii) without pain — ? pilocarpine.
(c) Efferent block: one pupil fails to respond to direct and consensual testing — consider third-nerve palsy.
(d) Complete afferent block: on shining light in affected eye *neither* pupil constricts; on shining light in fellow eye *both* pupils constrict normally.
(e) Relative afferent block: direct and consensual responses present in each eye but on swinging the flashlight from the fellow eye to the affected eye *both* pupils dilate. Afferent blocks, whether complete or relative, indicate optic nerve disease or whole retina disease.

## Ophthalmoscopy

Adequate visualisation of the fundus requires a darkened room and

**Figure 10.2:** The swinging flashlight test

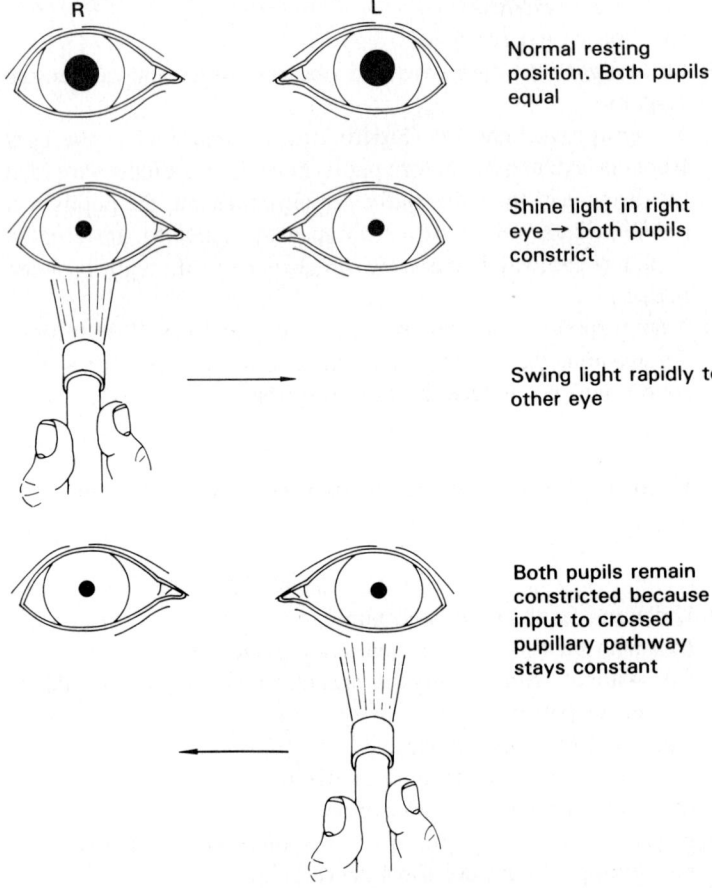

Normal resting position. Both pupils equal

Shine light in right eye → both pupils constrict

Swing light rapidly to other eye

Both pupils remain constricted because input to crossed pupillary pathway stays constant

dilation of the pupil (mydriasis). Use tropicamide 0.5% available in single-dose Minims to dilate all pupils except in drowsy or unconscious patients or in any patient with a head injury. It acts in 10 minutes and lasts 2 to 4 hours.

The risk of provoking acute closed angle glaucoma with this drug is negligible.

**Visual fields**

The following screening method will pick up all gross visual field

*Left relative afferent pupil block* due to left optic neuritis, for example. Direct and consensual responses are present in each eye but on swinging flashlight test:

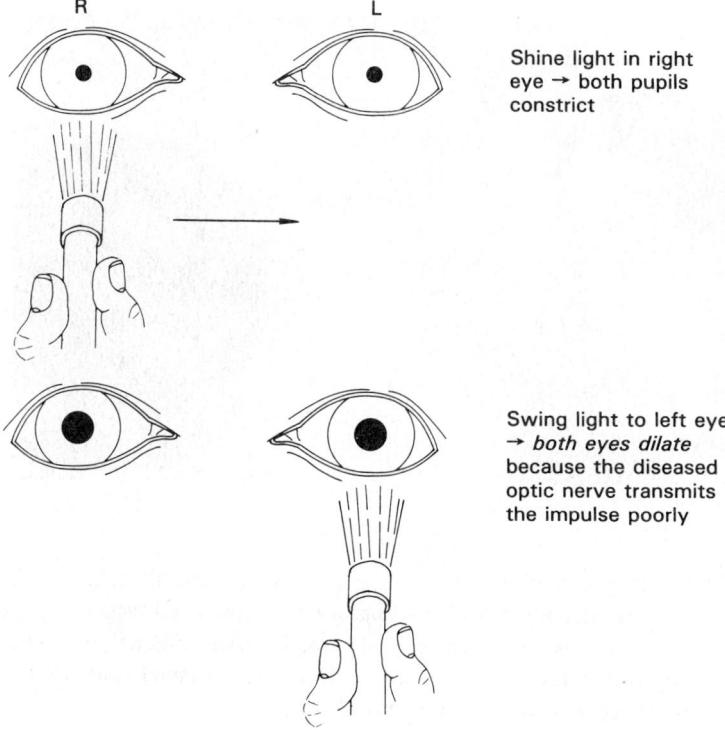

Shine light in right eye → both pupils constrict

Swing light to left eye → *both eyes dilate* because the diseased optic nerve transmits the impulse poorly

defects, these being the usual type associated with acute neurological disease. Specialist equipment is required to pick up small or relative defects such as are seen in chronic open angle glaucoma. In neurological disease, by and large, 'if a field defect is "equivocal", then it probably doesn't exist'.

(1) All four quadrants. Use the palms of your hands. They present large stationary targets and cause much less confusion. Test with both eyes open and then each eye separately, with the patient covering his or her fellow eye (Figure 10.3).

(2) Perimetry. Bring your open hands slowly in from the periphery until seen to outline the perimeter of the field. Waving fingers of hand provides unwanted additional clues.

**Figure 10.3:** Testing the visual fields: a screening method

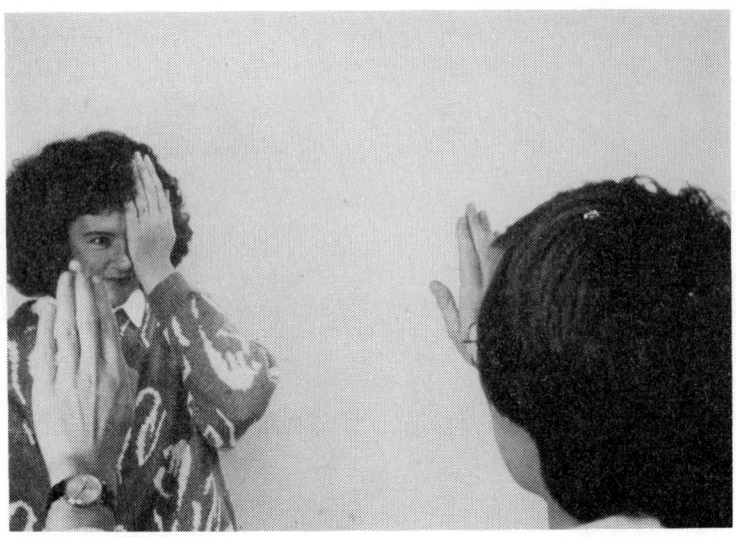

(3) Central sensation. The presence of a central scotoma is associated with loss of red sensation. Show a red target (e.g. a red pen top) to each eye separately. An affected eye will appreciate the colour as grey, orange or washed out; such a response indicates optic nerve disease.

Figure 10.4 shows common visual field defects and their differential diagnosis.

Optic atrophy occurs 6 weeks or later after a neurological event in the visual pathway. It is *not* a sign of acute disease, rather of a disease that was acute 6 weeks ago or longer (Figure 10.5).

## DIFFERENTIAL DIAGNOSIS

The simplest way to classify visual loss is by whether it is unilateral or bilateral, transient or persistent and whether the eye is red or not. Where possible, diagnoses are given in order of frequency with the commonest first.

**Figure 10.4:** Common visual field defects and their differential diagnoses

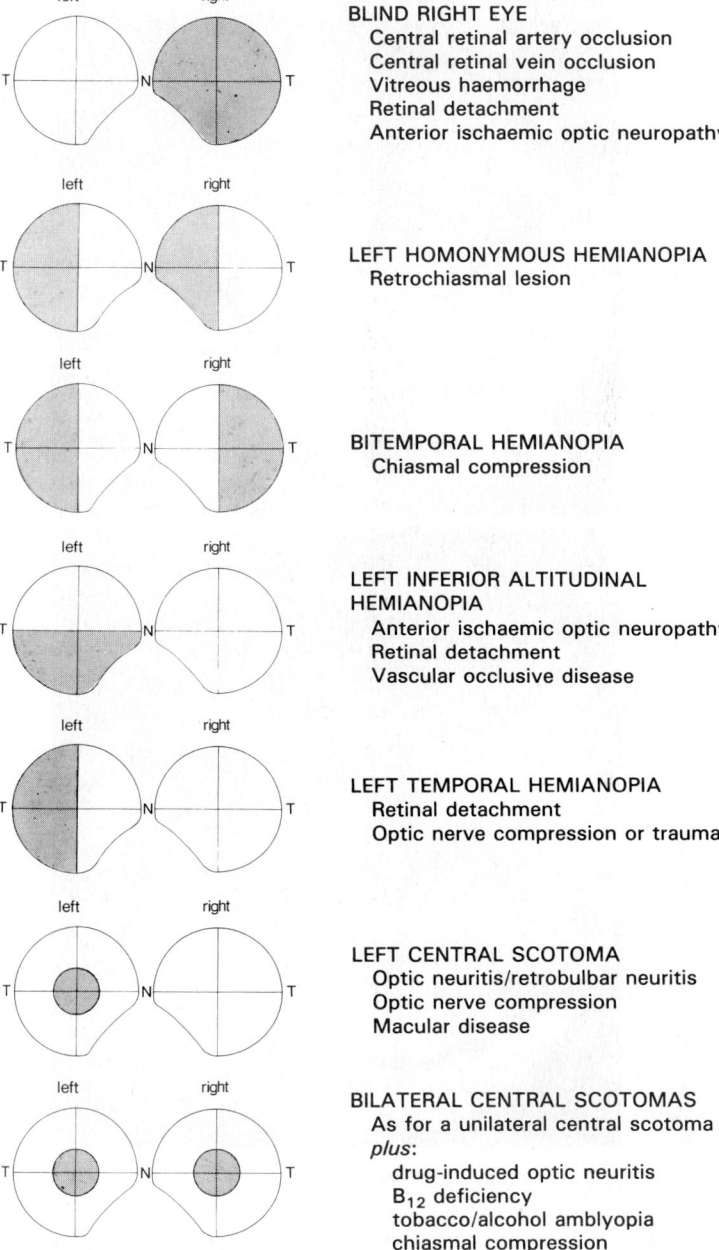

**BLIND RIGHT EYE**
Central retinal artery occlusion
Central retinal vein occlusion
Vitreous haemorrhage
Retinal detachment
Anterior ischaemic optic neuropathy

**LEFT HOMONYMOUS HEMIANOPIA**
Retrochiasmal lesion

**BITEMPORAL HEMIANOPIA**
Chiasmal compression

**LEFT INFERIOR ALTITUDINAL HEMIANOPIA**
Anterior ischaemic optic neuropathy
Retinal detachment
Vascular occlusive disease

**LEFT TEMPORAL HEMIANOPIA**
Retinal detachment
Optic nerve compression or trauma

**LEFT CENTRAL SCOTOMA**
Optic neuritis/retrobulbar neuritis
Optic nerve compression
Macular disease

**BILATERAL CENTRAL SCOTOMAS**
As for a unilateral central scotoma
*plus*:
    drug-induced optic neuritis
    $B_{12}$ deficiency
    tobacco/alcohol amblyopia
    chiasmal compression

181

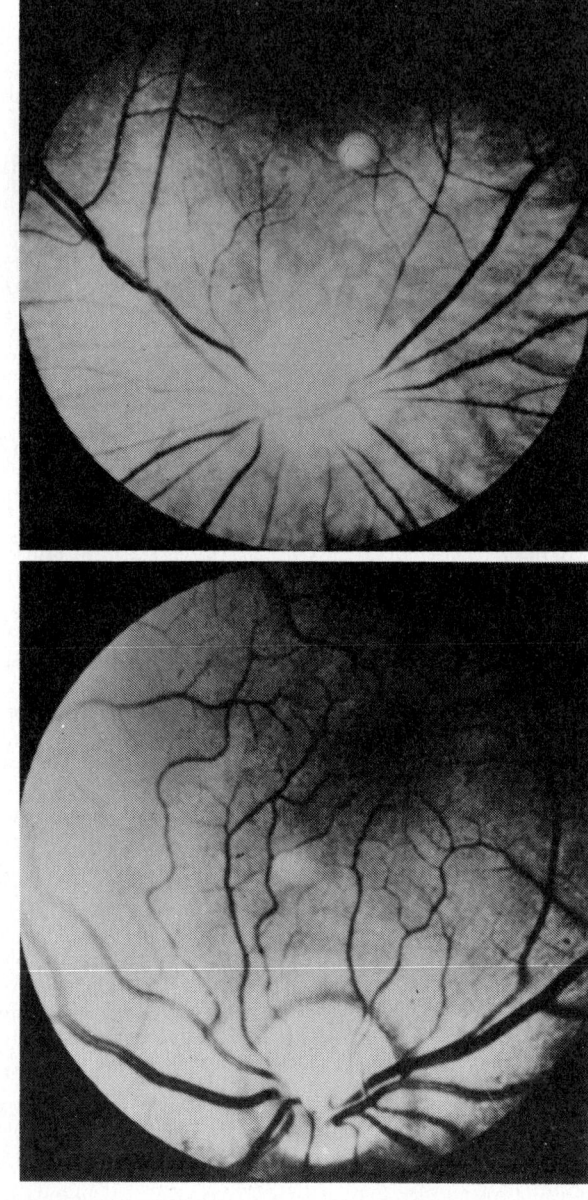

Figure 10.5: The normal disc (left) compared with the pale disc of optic atrophy (right)

## A. Unilateral and persistent

*Red and painful*

All too often, this is diagnosed as 'conjunctivitis' by the non-specialist; the clues are the severity of the pain and the impaired visual acuity.

(1) *Acute closed angle glaucoma*. Sudden painful loss of vision over a few minutes occurs, with corneal oedema, redness, a fixed dilated pupil and a rock-hard globe (compare the patient's ocular pressure with your own). Patients are acutely ill with nausea and vomiting and are often admitted to general surgical wards. It is the commonest ophthalmic cause of a laparotomy!

(2) Acute anterior uveitis. Sudden painful loss of vision over a few hours occurs with a fixed constricted pupil, redness and keratic precipitates sometimes visible as small white dots on the internal surface of the cornea. Occasionally pus is present in the anterior chamber, which can settle inferiorly to form a hypopyon.

*White and painless*

Apart from the last two, in all the following conditions the visual acuity suddenly drops to finger counting (CF) or worse.

(1) Central retinal artery occlusion (Figure 10.6). The vision goes out like a light to hand movements (HM) or worse. Signs include: complete afferent pupil defect; thin, tortuous retinal vessels sometimes with 'cattletrucking' of red cells; pale, oedematous retina; cherry-red macula. Emergency treatment if instituted within 30 minutes may result in complete recovery of vision when the cause is embolic. Intravenous acetazolamide (500 mg), ocular massage (press on the eye to reduce intraocular pressure) and 5% $CO_2$ in $O_2$ (breathing into a paper bag) are all effective and mandatory. Determination of erythrocyte sedimentation rate (ESR) is essential in all cases to exclude giant cell arteritis.

(2) Central retinal vein occlusion (Figure 10.7). The vision fails more slowly like a light being dimmed to 6/60 or CF. Signs include: complete afferent pupil defect; multiple retinal haemorrhages and cotton wool spots; dilated, tortuous veins; disc oedema. Do not confuse with papilloedema in which the visual acuity is normal or near normal and any haemorrhages are adjacent to the disc only.

183

**Figure 10.6:** Central retinal artery occlusion

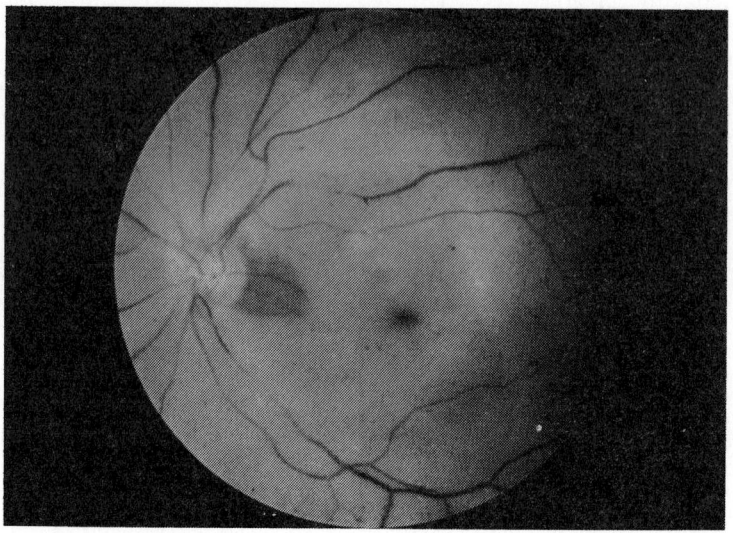

(3) Retinal detachment (Figure 10.8). A detachment may be preceded by flashing lights or floaters in one quadrant followed by an increasing field defect experienced as 'a curtain being drawn over the eye', which eventually obscures central vision. Ophthalmosopy shows a detached retina but only when large.

It is difficult to exclude a small or peripheral retinal detachment without specialist equipment, and so a history of recent onset of floaters requires an ophthalmic referral.

(4) *Vitreous haemorrhage.* No red reflex or fundal view can be obtained even when the pupil has been dilated and the lens is clear. Commonest causes are diabetes and retinal detachment.

(5) *Macular haemorrhage* (Figure 10.9). Senile macular degeneration may progress suddenly to a haemorrhagic disciform degeneration. A large macular haemorrhage is visible on ophthalmoscopy.

(6) *Anterior ischaemic optic neuropathy* (Figure 10.10). Sudden loss of vision to finger counting or worse occurs *or* there is sudden development of an attitudinal hemianopia (Figure 10.4). There is usually a complete afferent pupil defect. Disc signs are variable, ranging from gross oedema to minimal changes in the surrounding nerve fibre layer. It is to be distinguished from

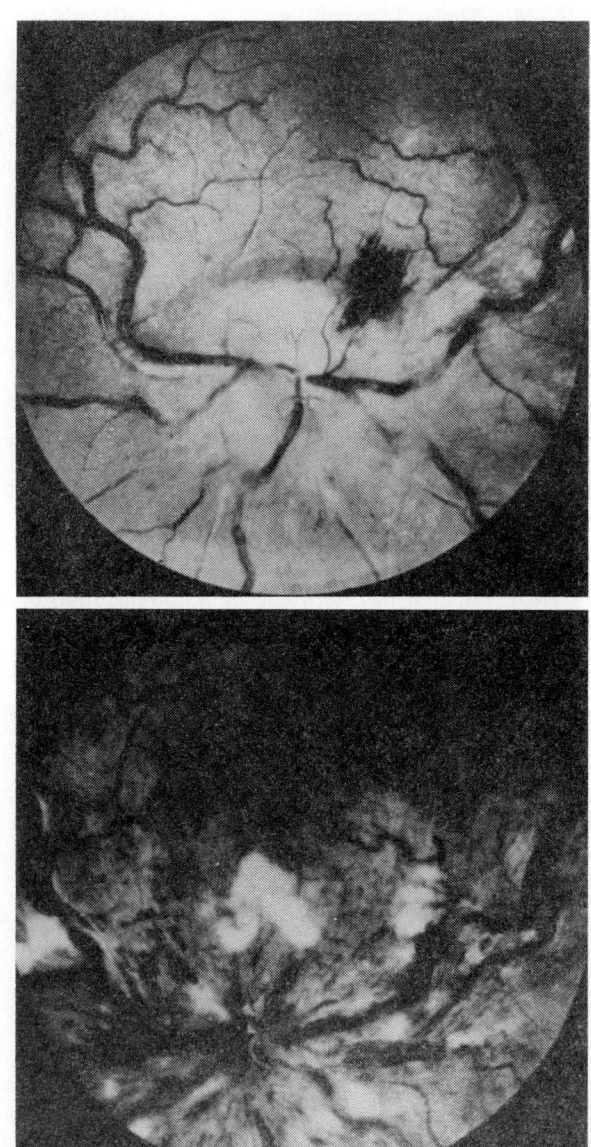

**Figure 10.7:** Central retinal vein occlusion (left) compared with acute papilloedema (right)

**Figure 10.8:** Inferior retinal detachment. This would cause a superior field defect

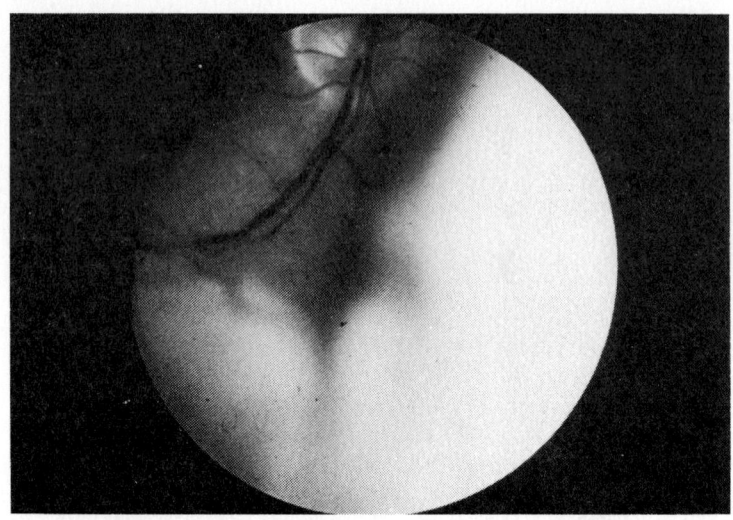

**Figure 10.9:** Macular haemorrhage as a complication of senile macular degeneration (haemorrhagic disciform macular degeneration)

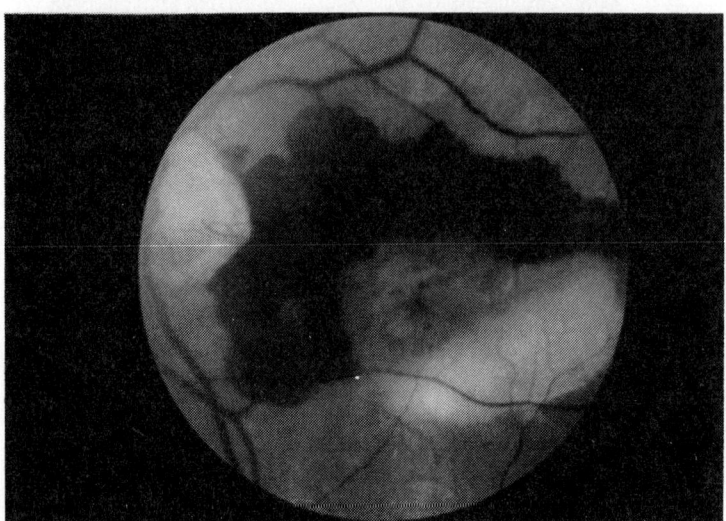

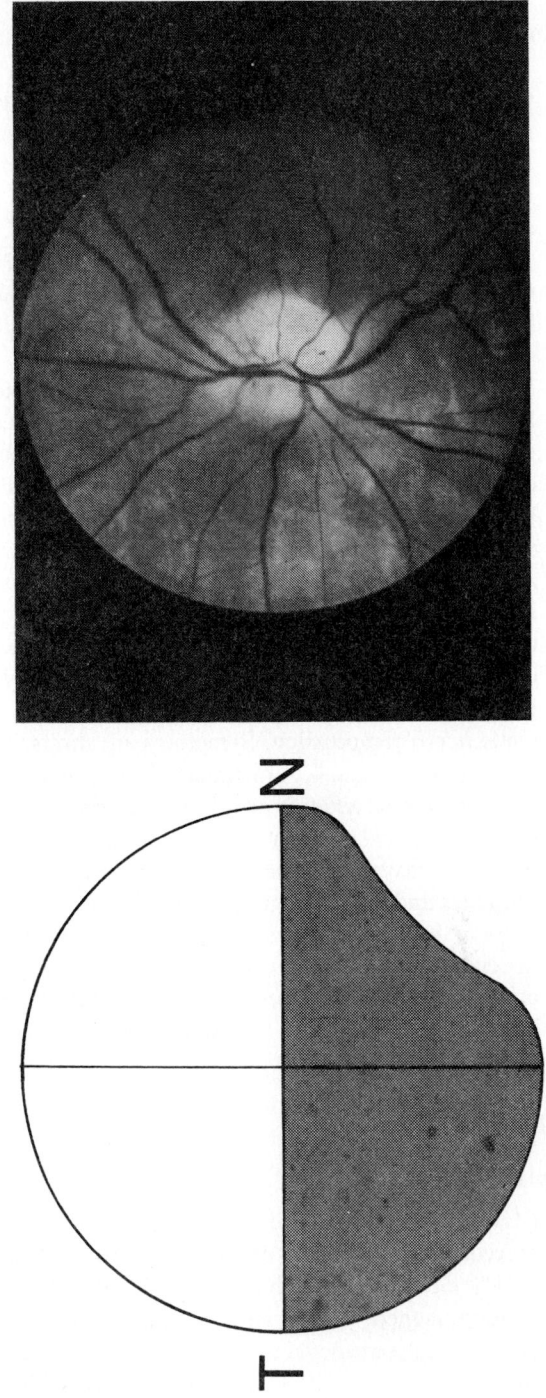

**Figure 10.10:** Anterior ischaemic optic neuropathy with inferior altitudinal hemianopia. Note oedema of superior half of disc

papilloedema in which *the vision stays good*. The most important cause is giant cell arteritis, and the ESR must be performed in all cases. General features of this disease include polymyalgia rheumatica, tender and non-pulsatile temporal arteries, jaw claudication, weight loss and malaise, though these are not necessarily present. Emergency treatment is necessary to protect the fellow eye which can lose vision in under 6 hours; immediate high dose IV steroids should be considered in all cases. Other causes include diabetes and atherosclerosis.

(7) *Retrobulbar neuritis (RBN)/optic neuritis.* Acute or subacute loss of vision in youth or middle age to variable degree (in mild cases visual acuity may be as good as 6/9 but when severe it may be reduced to no perception of light (NPL)). Be particularly suspicious in a patient who complains of poor vision and has a visual acuity of 6/4, 6/6; the 6/6 eye may have RBN. Signs are: *relative* afferent pupil block; reduced red sensation; central scotoma; normal fundus. The fellow eye may show optic atrophy as evidence of past involvement. The patient may ·complain of pain in the affected eye on eye movement, especially on extremes of gaze.

(8) Optic nerve compression. Symptoms are similar to RBN but the onset is more gradual, sometimes with development of unilateral field defects in addition to central scotoma. The disc may be oedematous and associated with retinal venous engorgement, though it may be normal. Look for associated signs such as proptosis and ocular motility disturbances. A CAT scan should show a large mass lesion responsible for the compression. Specialised views of the orbit, contrast cisternography and even craniotomy are sometimes indicated if compression is suspected but cannot be ruled out by simpler tests.

## B. Bilateral and transient

*Migraine*

(1) *Classical migraine.* The field defect is usually bilateral and precedes the headache. It usually starts centrally and works slowly out to the periphery over 10–20 minutes with a scintillating, jagged, leading edge; it usually looks like the fortifications around a medieval town and hence is called a 'fortification spectrum' (Figure 10.11). It may occur without subsequent headache and is· then termed *acephalgic migraine*. Occasionally

**Figure 10.11**: Development over time of a scintillating scotoma or 'fortification spectrum' in classical migraine

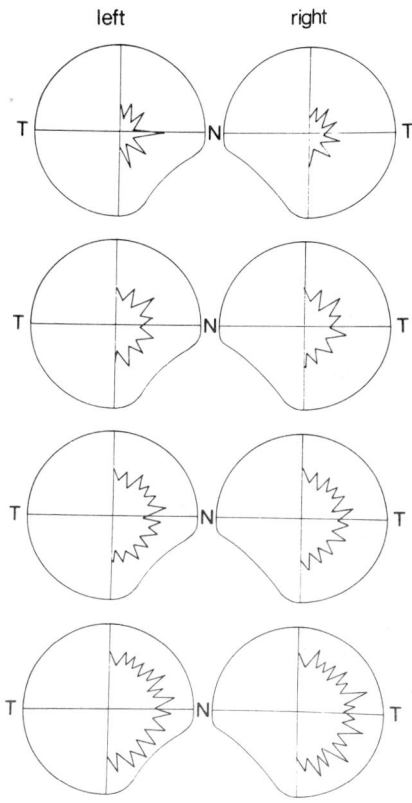

there may be transient complete blindness.

(2) *Basilar migraine*. Bilateral loss of vision, which is more usually blurring than complete, occurs over a few seconds to minutes in young women. No fortification spectra are seen. There are associated brainstem signs such as altered consciousness, ataxia, dysarthria, vertigo, paraesthesiae around the mouth, tongue and lips and weakness of sensory loss in any or all four limbs.

*Vertebrobasilar TIA*

These occur in older patients, usually over 50, with a sudden onset of bilateral loss or blurring of vision and with at least one but preferably more of the following: diplopia, slurred speech, ataxia,

189

hemiparesis, quadriparesis, hemisensory/all four limb sensory disturbance. Blurred vision or dizziness as the only symptom is not sufficient to make the diagnosis.

### Papilloedema

Transient obscurations may be bilateral.

## C. Unilateral and transient

### Amaurosis fugax

The term means 'transient blindness' but should be restricted to uniocular episodes of transient loss of vision lasting several seconds or minutes without headache. Patients often describe a grey/black shutter coming down over the vision of one eye. It is only a symptom, *not* a diagnosis, and usually indicates transient ischaemic attacks (TIA) in the affected eye.

The usual cause is microemboli (platelets, fibrin, thrombus or cholesterol crystals) from carotid artery atheroma or from the heart entering the retinal circulation. Reduced ocular blood flow due to a very tight internal carotid stenosis is an infrequent cause. There may be associated symptoms of cerebral ischaemia such as dysphasia or contralateral hemiparesis. Listen to the carotid artery for a bruit and examine the heart. Within 5 years about 35% will have died or had a stroke.

Although this is the commonest variety of transient unilateral loss of vision, the treatable conditions described below should *always* be considered. Once ocular causes have been ruled out, patients should be referred to a neurologist and assessed for carotid angiography or surgery. It is reasonable to start all patients on aspirin 300 mg daily.

### Migrainous unilateral visual loss

Migrainous visual disturbances usually affect *both* eyes. Rarely migraine can affect one eye only (see section on migraine). It is distinguishable from TIA because of the usual association with headache and the *slowly evolving, positive* visual phenomena.

### Papilloedema

Transient obscurations of vision (episodes of sudden blindness or blurring of vision) can occur in patients with papilloedema (Figure 10.7). The attacks are usually precipitated by bending over. Ophthalmoscopy will reveal the papilloedema, which can be distinguished from other causes of disc oedema because it is *usually bilateral* and the vision is *good*. The presence of obscurations means that emergency referral to a neurologist/neurosurgeon is essential.

### Giant cell arteritis

An impending optic nerve infarct (see section on anterior ischaemic optic neuropathy) can cause transient loss of vision.

### Impending central retinal artery occlusion

Look for anaemia, polycythaemia and leukaemia.

### Intermittent closed angle glaucoma

Associations are pain in the affected eye with a pressure rise during the attack. Haloes may occur and the vision is blurred rather than completely lost. It often proceeds to an irreversible attack. If there is any doubt about the diagnosis, an ophthalmologist's opinion should be sought.

## D. Bilateral and persistent

This is the least common variety of acute visual failure. The commonest cause is a unilateral acute loss of vision in the presence of pre-existing disease in the fellow eye such as cataract or macular degeneration, or end-stage disease in both eyes such as chronic open angle glaucoma or retinitis pigmentosa.

### Optic neuritis

(1) *Demyelination.* Simultaneous bilateral retrobulbar neuritis is very uncommon; the more frequent pattern is for the eyes to be affected sequentially.
(2) *Drugs.* Chloroquine, quinine, ethambutol, chloramphenicol, the oral contraceptive pill, disulphiram, digoxin.

### Tobacco/alcohol amblyopia/B12 deficiency

Both of these cause a central scotoma which involves the blind spot (centrocaecal scotoma) but this is clinically indistinguishable on simple testing from a true central scotoma. Serum B12 estimation should be performed on all cases of suspected optic nerve disease.

### Cortical blindness

The hallmark of this condition is that the pupillary light reactions are *normal*, since the cortex does not participate in the reflex arc. The commonest cause is bilateral occipital lobe infarction due to atheromatous disease or severe hypotension from any cause (it may be seen after overaggressive treatment of hypertension). The sudden onset will give a clue, and signs are total blindness or bilateral constricted fields (tunnel vision).

### Chiasmal compression

A rare cause of acute visual loss. It usually presents as gradual loss of vision with optic atrophy, bitemporal hemianopia or central scotomata. Causes are pituitary tumour, craniopharyngioma and chiasmal glioma.

### Hysteria

This must always be a diagnosis of exclusion made after thorough investigation for organic causes.

## ACUTE DIPLOPIA

Acute onset diplopia may represent a neurological emergency. At the very least it engenders a lot of anxiety in both patient and doctor. Below are listed, in order of commonness, the conditions which should be considered.

## Uniocular diplopia

It is distinguished from binocular diplopia by not being abolished when the fellow eye is covered. Patients are often labelled hysterical but this is in fact an exceedingly rare variety of ocular hysteria. Causes are local and include cataract, keratoconus, subluxated lens, macular disease, excessive lacrimation and blocked tear ducts.

## Binocular diplopia

The diplopia is abolished by covering either eye. Always look for other neurological signs before deciding on the diagnosis.

### Adult consecutive divergent squint

The commonest cause of adult onset diplopia is the progression from

192

a childhood convergent squint through a 'straight' period to a divergent state. The onset of divergence is heralded by at first intermittent then constant horizontal diplopia.

## VIth nerve palsy

Patients complain of horizontal diplopia on looking to the side of the paretic lateral rectus. Examination shows that the affected eye fails to abduct past the midline. In the absence of associated neurological signs a VIth nerve palsy is relatively benign. Vascular lesions and diabetes mellitus are by far the commonest causes, with tumour, trauma, demyelination and middle ear infections making up the remainder.

## IVth nerve palsy

The affected muscle is the superior oblique which is responsible for depressing the eye in adduction (the muscle of reading) and so patients complain of vertical diplopia on reading and on looking down at a flight of stairs or a kerb. The ocular motility defect may be difficult to recognise and so the history is the most important diagnostic tool. This is the commonest cranial nerve palsy after blunt trauma to the head; other causes are vascular lesions, diabetes mellitus and rarely tumour.

## IIIrd nerve palsy

Classically the eye is turned down and out and there is ptosis and pupillary dilation. Any diplopia is often blocked by the ptotic lid. The most important cause is aneurysm of the posterior communicating artery with diabetes mellitus, vascular, tumour, trauma and giant cell arteritis making up most of the remainder.

Posterior communicating artery aneurysm is *painful* and shows *pupillary involvement*; diabetic IIIrd nerve palsies tend to spare the pupil but may be painful. A IIIrd nerve palsy that is painful and involves the pupil in the absence of trauma is due to an aneurysm *until proved otherwise*. The ESR must also always be checked to help exclude giant cell arteritis.

## Ophthalmoplegic migraine

Onset is nearly always before the age 10 with usually an already established history of migraine. The ophthalmoplegia is transient, lasting for days to weeks with associated headaches at onset, and is most frequently a IIIrd nerve palsy. It is a diagnosis of exclusion and is made at peril until all other causes of cranial nerve palsy have been thoroughly investigated.

## Myasthenia gravis (MG)

Any patient with an apparent IVth or VIth nerve palsy or a IIIrd nerve palsy with normal pupils may have MG. Similarly consider MG if the pattern of ocular motility disturbance does not fit with a single cranial nerve palsy or is bilateral or the ptosis is variable. Symptoms and signs of generalised limb, bulbar and respiratory muscle weakness may give additional pointers.

Diagnosis is usually established by a history of fatiguability and by a Tensilon (Edrophonium) test. False negative or equivocal responses are not uncommon and should be rechecked. The test should always be performed with the patient lying on a couch in the presence of another doctor with resuscitation equipment available. Be especially cautious in patients with obstructive airways and/or cardiac disease. Give a 0.1 mg test dose followed by 5 mg *only*. Atropine (0.6 mg IV) should be given if bradycardia develops. All patients with suspected MG should be assessed by a neurologist.

## Dysthyroid eye disease

Dysthyroid eye disease may present as acute onset diplopia and because of its frequency should always be considered. Look for other signs of ocular involvement such as lid retraction, lid lag and exophthalmos. The ocular motility disturbance is most often a failure of elevation due to inferior rectus involvement but may be bizarre. Biochemical investigation of thyroid function often gives normal results.

**ACKNOWLEDGEMENT**

We are indebted to Mr C.H. Mody for the preparation of the illustrations.

**FURTHER READING**

Coakes, R.L. and Holmes-Sellors, D. (1985) *An Outline of Ophthalmology*, Wright, Bristol

Glaser, J. (1978) *Neuro-ophthalmology*, Harper & Row, Hagerstown, MD

Kanski, J.J. (1984) *Ophthalmology colour aids*, Churchill Livingstone, Edinburgh

Miller, N.R. (Ed.) (1985) *Walsh & Hoyt's Clinical Neuro-opthalmology*, 4th edn, Williams & Wilkins, Baltimore, MD

# 11

# Spinal Cord Injury and Spinal Cord Compression

Gordon F.G. Findlay

## INTRODUCTION

The presentation of the multitude of diseases which can affect the spinal cord, the cauda equina and the intraspinal nerve roots can be of very insidious onset, but more often they present as a rapidly progressing problem requiring urgent evaluation and treatment. The time course of some of the pathologies which cause cord compression can indeed be very acute, as in the case of an acute extradural abscess, but more usually the pathology has been present for some time prior to the actual onset of the neurological deficit. As such pathological processes progress, they increasingly compromise the integrity of the spinal cord until such time as the normal compensating mechanisms available to the cord are exhausted. At that stage neurological deficit can appear suddenly and deteriorate with alarming speed.

No matter what the actual pathology may be, it is true to say that probably the most important factor to influence the outcome of treatment is the severity of the neurological deficit at the time of presentation. The more marked the deficit has become, the less good are the chances of management being successful in restoring normal cord function, and moreover, the risks of surgery in particular are often considerably increased. It can readily be appreciated that it is of the utmost importance, therefore, to make the diagnosis of spinal cord compression at the earliest possible moment. Unfortunately, it is then that the diagnosis may be least obvious. Diagnosis at that stage can only be achieved by a great awareness of the possibility and along with this must go the realisation of the need for prompt action when the diagnosis is considered.

It is an unfortunate fact that the diagnosis of a neurological emergency is often surrounded by a sense of mystique among clinicians who do not encounter such problems routinely. It is certainly true that it is an exacting task to define accurately the nature of any pathological process causing cord compression as the range of such pathologies is enormous. Fortunately, there is a considerable degree of similarity in the way in which these diseases present and, therefore, it is not too difficult to come to the more overall diagnosis of spinal cord compression. Indeed, in relation to the clinician seeing such a patient at the first presentation, the diagnosis of spinal cord compression is all that has to be made. It is the clinicians responsible for the definitive treatment who are required to come to the exact pathological diagnosis prior to therapy, and therefore this chapter will concentrate on how to make a diagnosis of cord or root compression rather than differentiating between the various underlying causes.

## PATHOPHYSIOLOGY

In order to appreciate the manifestations of the clinical syndrome of spinal compression, some basic understanding of the underlying processes involved is necessary. The spinal column and the tissues it contains consist of a wide variety of structures which can be affected by pathological processes leading ultimately to the development of neurological deficit. It is easiest to consider these by reference to a cross-section of the canal as shown in Figure 11.1.

The spinal column itself gives rise to the most common pathologies that lead to cord compression. The commonest disease to affect the spinal column and to cause cord compression is degenerative disease. Cervical spondylosis is widespread in the community and is invariably present, at least radiologically, in people aged over 70 years. Cervical spondylotic myelopathy is probably the commonest cause of cord compression treated in a neurosurgical unit as spondylotic change is so prevalent. However, actual myelopathy is in fact a rare feature of this disease, with only a small minority of those affected by cervical spondylosis developing this complication. The onset of myelopathy is only rarely acute in the absence of superimposed trauma. Acute cervical disc rupture can occur and in this case rapid neurological deficit can ensue. Degenerative disease affecting the thoracic spine is much less common, but thoracic disc protrusion can cause some of the most severe examples of cord compression. Although the pathological

**Figure 11.1:** Cross-section of the neural canal

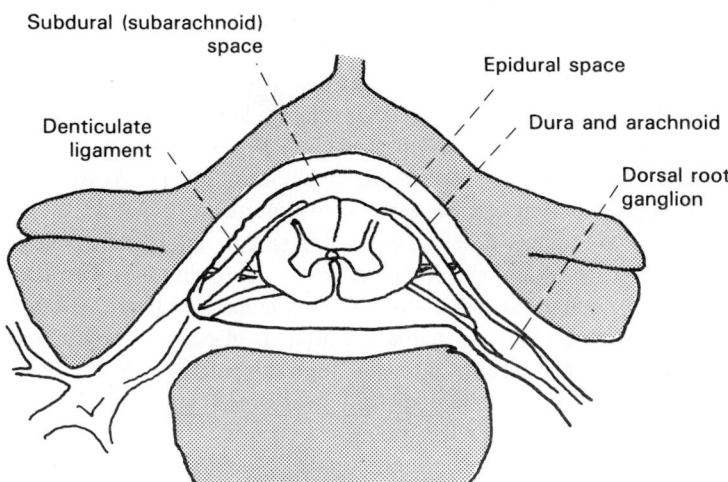

process here usually takes years to develop, neurological deterioration in the later stages may be very acute.

The commonest pathology that affects the spinal skeleton and leads to cord compression presenting acutely is metastatic involvement of the vertebra, usually starting in the vertebral body or in the pedicle. Cord compression is due to the extension of tumour out of the vertebra itself such that the extradural space is encroached upon and the cord is displaced and finally compressed. On other occasions, the metastatic disease in the body may so weaken the spine that deformity due to collapse occurs and the cord becomes angulated and compressed. There is also good evidence that thrombosis of important end arteries to the cord can occur and may account for some of the reasons why the deficit can be irreversible despite adequate therapy. On rare occasions, pathological fracture can occur leading to very dramatic onset of pain and neurological deficit. Obviously, any of the primary bone tumours can affect the spine but these are fortunately rare, unless one considers haematological tumours such as lymphoma or myeloma to be genuinely primary tumours.

Spinal osteomyelitis is an unusual rather than rare disease. Even today, in developed societies, the commonest infection is tuberculosis;

197

a disease by no means confined to immigrant populations. Other organisms, such as staphylococci, *E. coli* and less commonly *Brucella*, cause somewhat more acute infections but, irrespective of organism, cord compression is due (as in tumours) to the mechanisms of invasion of the extradural space, spinal deformity and infarction. Such infections develop relatively slowly and the presentation is usually of a subacute type. However, again, once the mechanisms of compensation are exhausted, the progress of the neurological deficit can be very rapid indeed.

There are many other processes that can affect the skeleton producing cord compression such as congenital deformities, metabolic bone disease and vascular anomalies. These are all rather unusual but present in a manner similar to that of other structural lesions of the vertebrae where, although the pathological process is of long standing, the final neurological presentation can be very rapid demanding urgent treatment.

Turning to the extradural space, pathological conditions restricted entirely to this space are relatively uncommon. As has been said above, neoplasms of the vertebrae often invade the extradural space but it is important to realise that, on occasion, blood-borne metastases may arise *de novo* in the extradural space and consequently only rarely show evidence of their presence on plain radiology. This is particularly true in the case of lymphomas. There are two conditions that affect the extradural space producing very acute neurological deficit. Although uncommon, they are both eminently treatable provided that the diagnosis is appreciated immediately. On the other hand, if diagnosis is delayed by only a few hours, severe irreversible neurological deficit ensues. These conditions are: acute extradural haematoma, which may be spontaneous or related to vascular anomalies or anticoagulant therapy; and acute extradural abscess. Both these conditions present with acute, very severe, spinal pain and paraspinal spasm, especially in cases of abscess. At that stage there may be no neurological deficit, but, if the diagnosis is not made by urgent myelography, complete paraplegia can develop within hours. Therefore, a high index of suspicion is required to diagnose such conditions.

The intradural space contains two 'compartments': the intradural extramedullary (subarachnoid) space and the intramedullary 'space'. There are a multitude of fairly rare lesions that arise in the extramedullary space but the commonest are neurofibromata and meningiomas. Fortunately, extramedullary lesions tend to present in fairly uniform manner and, although usually of fairly long standing, their final neurological presentation can be very rapid. It is not easy to differentiate clinically between extradural and intradural cord compression, and this often requires specialist neuroradiology. However, again the important diagnosis to make is that of cord compression itself, leading to appropriate specialist referral.

In the intramedullary compartment, there are again many different pathological processes that can occur. Some of these, such as the glial neoplasms, arteriovenous malformations and syringomyelia, require neurosurgical treatment, but many of these diseases are neurological, such as demyelination and transverse myelitis. Although there are often clues which in expert hands can differentiate between neurological and surgical cord diseases, one can never be certain about this and such patients still require urgent referral for neuroradiological investigation to allow the exclusion of a surgically correctable lesion. Indeed, even patients who are already known to have a disease such as multiple sclerosis may occasionally develop acute cord dysfunction due to another more treatable cause such as acute cervical disc prolapse.

Having broadly considered the types of pathology that can produce acute spinal neurological deficit, some attention has to be paid to the effects which such pathological processes produce at different levels of the spinal canal. It may seem obvious to state that pathology in the cervical spine is likely to produce a neurological picture which affects both the upper and lower limbs. However, this is not always true and, especially with anterior midline lesions, the only neurological deficit may be in the lower limbs. Below the cervical spine it can be very difficult to determine a motor level between T1 and T12, as in such lesions all muscle groups in the legs will be affected and accurate localisation of a level depends almost exclusively on sensory examination. Below L1/2 a major change occurs as, of course, in the adult the spinal cord stops at this level. Therefore, below L1/2 lesions will produce abnormalities of the cauda equina rather than of the cord. Such patients will present with lower rather than upper motor signs.

## CLINICAL FEATURES

There is really very little difficulty in making a diagnosis of spinal cord compression when there is already marked neurological deficit. However, as has been said already, one of the most important factors affecting the outcome of therapy is the extent of the deficit present at the time of treatment. It is imperative that the diagnosis of acute neurological involvement of the spine is appreciated at the earliest possible stage and, ideally, prior to the onset of neurological involvement. Obviously this ideal is unattainable in many instances but there are situations where such a diagnosis can be made. For example, in metastatic cord compression, pain is often present for some days or weeks prior to the onset of neurological deficit. If a patient with a known malignancy presents initially with only spinal pain (see below), then plain radiology at that point in time may well show the metastatic vertebral involvement. Treatment with radiotherapy at this stage dramatically reduces the likelihood of the future development of neurological deficit, so avoiding the problem altogether.

Although early diagnosis is not easy, it is fortunate that patients presenting with cord compression tend to do so in a fairly typical fashion regardless of the actual pathological cause. The presentation consists of a constellation of symptoms and signs referrable to pain and to sensory, motor and sphincteric function. Although the time course and previous history may vary considerably, the association of this constellation of symptoms should at the very least lead to a presumed diagnosis of spinal cord disease.

## Pain

Pain is frequently the first symptom to appear in spinal disease. The duration of this symptom varies widely and may have been present for years as in a case of cervical spondylotic myelopathy, or may be of sudden onset as in acute extradural abscess. Pain may be absent in some cases such as transverse myelitis, but the absence of pain does not imply the absence of a surgically treatable lesion. Pain is typically experienced at the site of the lesion and may have several associated features. Pain associated with structural disease such as a metastasis is usually continuous, though the severity may fluctuate. It is often exacerbated by moving or coughing and straining, and, on the contrary is relieved by lying down. Where marked spinal deformity and instability are present, the pain can be agonising and only partially relieved by lying completely still, the slightest movement causing pain.

Back pain is, of course, one of the most common symptoms presenting to a general practitioner and it is very difficult to pick out the patient whose complaint of back pain represents more sinister pathology at a stage prior to the development of neurological signs. However, a history of pain which is severe and unremitting should alert suspicion as the vast majority of patients with mechanical back pain have a fluctuating history with good as well as bad spells. Spinal pain in a child or adolescent should always be considered as being significant. This is especially true if it is associated with paraspinal muscle spasm and if the pain is worse at night, as these factors make the likelihood of an intramedullary tumour very high. A complaint of spinal pain in a patient who is known to have had a primary neoplasm elsewhere should also be taken seriously. In passing, however, it should be noted that over half of the patients who present with metastatic cord compression have no evidence of a primary tumour at the time of presentation. The absence of a known primary, therefore, should not preclude the diagnosis of metastatic cord compression.

Diseases that affect and compress the intraspinal nerve roots, as well as the cord such as cervical spondylosis may cause the typical pain of root involvement. This is a sharp shooting pain which radiates down the path of the root. Thus, in the neck, root involvement causes pain radiating down the arm into the hand; in the thoracic area, it causes typical girdle pain; and in the lumbar area, it causes root pain or sciatica in the leg. The presence of root pain strongly indicates pathology in the spine.

Another type of pain suggestive of a spinal origin is the type of pain which comes from the involvement of the cord itself. Such pain is more nebulous and harder to describe. It is often felt as a deep, burning sensation experienced in a more regional manner than root pain. Thus it may affect a whole limb rather than having a radicular distribution. If the patient has marked hypertonicity in the lower limbs, this in itself may be painful, and feelings of tightness around the knees or even a bursting sensation in the muscles of the leg may be reported.


## Sensory symptoms

The first symptom to occur when neurological deficit appears is often that of altered sensation. In the case of cord compression, the patient typically develops numbness starting in the feet and then ascending higher until the level of the lesion is reached. Many different descriptions of such sensations are used by patients, who often employ such terms as 'coldness', 'cotton wool' or 'deadness'.

They may even misinterpret sensory symptoms and describe them as weakness. Involvement of a root tends to give a more localised problem presenting with tingling and paraesthesiae, which in themselves may be painful.

Disturbance of the posterior columns leads to sensory deficit but here patients tend not to interpret such deficits as sensory. Rather, they will complain of difficulty in walking or balance. Where there is marked involvement of the spinothalamic tracts, the patient may notice disturbance of temperature sensation. Typically, this is noticed when testing the temperature of bath water. The finding of reduced pain and temperature sensation in one limb associated with weakness in the other constitutes the Brown–Séquard syndrome, strongly indicating cord disease.

In some situations sensory loss can be so severe that the patients can burn themselves without noticing. The finding of burn marks and associated trophic changes of the skin suggests this and in the upper limbs strongly suggests a diagnosis of syringomyelia. In patients with cervical disease, flexion of the neck may cause unpleasant sensory symptoms which radiate downwards rather like an electric shock. This Lhermitte's sign is sometimes misconstrued to be diagnostic of demyelinating disease but it should be appreciated that it can occur in any pathology affecting the cervical cord.

## Motor symptoms

Little requires to be said about motor symptoms as they tend to produce quite obvious deficits. However, it has to be appreciated that, although it is much easier to diagnose cord compression once marked weakness has ensued, in almost all instances the chances of recovery following treatment are markedly affected by the severity of the weakness. Thus, the onset of weakness has to be recognised immediately, allowing early referral and therapy.

The earliest symptoms of weakness in the lower limbs tend to be those of gait disturbance with a feeling of unsteadiness, a tendency to drag the feet and scuff the toes and frequent falls. Following this it becomes difficult to climb stairs and then ambulation even on the flat becomes impossible. At this stage, the patient has to hold on to pieces of furniture to get across the room, and it is only a short step to the stage when the patient can no longer weight-bear and is confined to bed.

At this stage, it should be noted that, although the patient can no longer walk, the term 'paraplegia' is only appropriate if there is absolutely no movement in the legs at all. If there is even only a little voluntary movement left, then the term 'paraparesis' should be used. This is of importance as in some conditions surgical treatment can be of little avail if paraplegia has been present for more than 24 hours. The differentiation of paraparesis from paraplegia is, therefore, of great importance.

## Sphincteric disturbance

The onset of sphincteric disturbance is usually a late feature of progressive cord of cauda equina compression. However, in the more acute types of compression, such as the rupture of a lumbar disc causing acute cauda equina compression, urinary retention may develop along with the other neurological deficits very quickly. The onset of bladder disturbance requires immediate recognition and treatment as retention present for greater than 24 hours has a dramatically reduced chance of recovery after decompression, even in the case of a benign lesion such as a disc prolapse.

Unfortunately, it is often the development of sphincter disturbance which eventually gives rise to the belated recognition of cord compression. Its presence in a patient with a paraparesis, say due to a metastasis, is usually a poor prognostic sign as it indicates severe cord compromise. However, even at this stage and provided the patient has not been totally paraplegic for too long, treatment can be effective if given quickly enough. This is particularly true in the case of lesions such as intradural meningiomas and neurofibromas, where treatment even in the face of paraplegia and retention can be effective due to the fact that such slowly growing lesions allow a greater amount of compensation in the cord than more aggressive lesions.

How then does one recognise sphincteric disturbance as being neurological? There are several clinical factors that can not only differentiate between obstructive rather than neurological retention but can also indicate whether, in the neurological case, the problem is that of an upper or lower motor neurone pathology. However, in the context of this text, the most important factor is whether retention is painful or not. Almost all examples of neurological retention are painless and result in a grossly distended bladder with overflow incontinence. Painless retention associated with any of the neurological symptoms mentioned above is almost always due to a neurological pathology affecting the cord or cauda equina. It can occur due to intracranial causes, but the absence of other symptoms and signs of spinal disease and the presence of other signs of cerebral dysfunction should make the diagnosis clear. Painless retention occasionally may be the only presenting problem of spinal disease, especially in sacral pathology. Therefore, the occurrence of painless retention should always be assumed to be neurological until proven otherwise.

Not all patients present in frank retention, and in such cases the differentiation of symptoms such as frequency, dribbling and hesitancy due to outflow or neurological problems is much more difficult. It is still safest to assume that the presence of such symptoms in association with other symptoms of spinal disease indicates a neurological cause.

## Examination

The examination of patients presenting with spinal disease is basically quite straightforward. It is much more difficult, and sometimes impossible, to differentiate clinically between the various causes of spinal neurological dysfunction without associated neuroradiological investigation. However, as has already been made clear, the important diagnosis to reach initially is that there is spinal cord compression and this is much more simple.

Examination of the spine is frequently omitted, perhaps because patients tend to be supine when examined. However, some very useful information can be gained and it must form part of every examination. Factors to look for include: obvious deformity such as a gibbus, indicating spinal deformity; cutaneous lesions such as naevi, indicating vascular anomalies, or sinuses suggesting congenital abnormalities; paravertebral masses, indicating infection or neoplastic invasion; and localised spinal tenderness.

Sensory examination consists of assessing the function of both the spinothalamic tracts and the posterior columns. Examination of the spinothalamic tracts is most easily achieved by testing pinprick sensation and determining a sensory level. Sensory levels can be very helpful in indicating the level of cord involvement, but it must be appreciated that, especially in intramedullary lesions, the sensory level may appear to be spuriously low. Levels to pinprick in the cervical and lumbar areas follow recognised dermatomal patterns in the same way as motor involvement and are discussed in greater detail in the section on spinal trauma. On the trunk a sensory level at the nipple line suggests a spinal level at T4; at the umbilicus T10; and at the groin T12/L1. Full examination of spinothalamic sensation also requires the assessment of temperature sensation. The posterior columns can be assessed by examination of vibration, proprioception and light touch sensations. Perhaps the most useful of these is proprioception, which should be assessed in the fingers as well as the toes.

Examination of the motor system is almost self-explanatory. It is obviously important to assess the degree of weakness present but it is equally important to assess which muscles are involved so that a motor level can be determined. This is relatively easy in the arms and the legs but is virtually impossible on the trunk where reliance has to be placed on sensory levels. In addition to assessing power, it is important to look for evidence of wasting or fasciculation in the affected muscles as such signs indicate a lower motor neurone lesion. Although the presence of widespread fasciculation and wasting in the absence of sensory symptoms strongly suggests the presence of motor neurone disease, it is still necessary for such a patient to undergo full neurological assessment in order to rule out a more treatable entity.

In addition to examining the motor system with the patient supine, it is essential to examine the gait assuming that the patient can still walk. It is surprisingly common in spinal disease to find relatively little neurological deficit on supine examination but to see gross disturbance of the gait when the patient is asked to walk. If the gait is not examined, the degree of neurological involvement can be grossly underestimated. It is important to realise that gait disturbance is not always due to spinal disease and can be due to intracranial problems, especially in the posterior fossa. However, the history and other signs present should allow this to be differentiated.

Having examined the motor and sensory systems, it is necessary to look for other signs that allow the differentiation of upper and lower motor neuronal damage as this will indicate whether the disease process is affecting the cord, nerve roots or both. Table 11.1 shows the signs that allow this discrimination. It is important to note that when a cord deficit develops rapidly there may not have been enough time for the signs of spasticity to have developed. Thus, the absence of signs such as increased tone, clonus and exaggerated reflexes does not rule out cord involvement in the acute stage. This is analogous to the situation in which a patient is admitted with an acute cerebrovascular accident and the hemiplegic arm is almost

**Table 11.1:** Differentiation of upper and lower motor neurone signs

| Sign | Upper | Lower |
|------|-------|-------|
| Reflexes | Increased | Decreased |
| Tone | Increased | Decreased |
| Clonus | Present | Absent |
| Plantars | Extensor | Flexor |
| Fasciculation | Absent | Present |
| Wasting | Absent | Present |

always flaccid during the initial stages.

Neurological examination is incomplete without full general examination. This will include examination of the abdomen to see whether there is an enlarged bladder consequent on urinary retention. While seeking evidence of any other disease process present, it is particularly important to look for any evidence of an unsuspected primary tumour.

## MANAGEMENT

It should be clear from the above discussion that the principal role of the primary physician in the management of acute spinal disease is to recognise the diagnosis of cord or root compression and then to refer the patient without delay to an appropriate centre where the necessary neuroradiological facilities exist for the precise diagnosis to be made. It cannot be stressed sufficiently that delay in this matter in a case with rapidly evolving neurological deficit not only severely reduces the chances of therapy regaining the neurological function that has been lost, but also often increases the risks of that therapy producing unwanted complications. Obviously some degree of clinical assessment needs to be employed to decide exactly how much of an emergency exists. On the one hand, a patient with a slowly developing cervical spondylotic myelopathy need not be transferred as an emergency, though it must be appreciated that unnecessary delay should be avoided as the best surgical results arise when patients are treated at a relatively early stage of their disease (assuming them to be deteriorating). On the other hand, a patient presenting with acute cord compression from a metastasis or an extradural abscess needs urgent transfer even if the deficit seems to have stopped progressing. If there is any doubt about the time scale of the progression of the neurological deficit, it is always safer to rely on transfer at an early stage.

There are certain general measures which should be undertaken prior to transfer. For example, it may be appropriate to give the patient analgesics if he or she is in pain, and the presence of an enlarged bladder demands catheterisation. It is often sensible to check that the patient is not grossly anaemic, and, if in retention, then it is sensible to check quickly on renal function. It is not appropriate to await the results of any other blood investigations such as liver function or acid phosphatase, though it is sensible to have taken these tests if appropriate so that the results can be forwarded when available.

If X-ray facilities are available, then it is sensible to perform a chest X-ray. This may show evidence of a primary bronchogenic tumour or of multiple metastases, either of which might imply that active management could be inappropriate. It is also necessary to take formal spinal radiographs. The chest X-ray is inadequate to show the thoracic spine, and formal thoracic films should always be taken. The spinal films should be looked at to see whether there is any evidence of the following: obvious primary neoplasia; congenital deformity; degenerative changes showing as osteophytes or perhaps disc calcification in the thoracic spine; osteomyelitis showing as collapse with loss of definition of the adjacent disc space; and evidence of metastases such as loss of a pedicle or vertebral collapse. A word of caution about the interpretation of vertebral collapse is necessary as it is sometimes erroneously taken to imply the presence of malignant disease. This is very far from the case as it may be due to a large number of other causes among which are: infection, congenital deformity, osteoporosis and trauma.

Having come to the decision that the patient has incipient cord compression, referral to a neurosurgical unit is usually appropriate. On occasions, however, when there is no doubt that the pathology is that of a metastatic cord compression in a patient with a known malignancy, it may be appropriate to refer direct to the radiotherapist. If it is certain that the diagnosis is not one of infection, then it is sensible to commence the patient on steroids by giving an intravenous loading dose of dexamethasone 12 mg. This will not prevent the development of neurological deficit but it does often slow down the rate at which the deficit develops. On some occasions it can in fact lead to an improvement in the degree of neurological deficit, but it should be stressed that such improvement will only be temporary.

Once the patient has arrived at the neurological unit and has been assessed, a myelogram will normally be performed, though increasing use is being made of spinal CT scanning and magnetic resonance. Myelography is sometimes performed in the general unit prior to transfer, but this practice should not be encouraged. The principal reasons for this are that it often takes longer to organise than in the specialist unit and that, in non-specialist hands, it is possible that important information may be missed. Further than this, the information seen on the actual radiographs taken is only part of the story and a great deal can be learned from the way in which the dye flows through the spinal column. This information is only available to the neurosurgeon if the investigation is performed in the neurosurgical unit. A rarer though more worrying reason for these investigations to be performed in specialist units is that a lumbar puncture performed below the level of a complete block can lead to acute neurological deterioration in the same way as patients with posterior fossa lesions can cone following lumbar puncture.

The wider availability of CT scanning does raise the possibility of inappropriate investigation if not properly utilised. Although lesions of the vertebrae themselves are well shown by this technique, it can be very difficult to display an intradural lesion on a plain CT scan as these lesions often require contrast enhancement or intrathecal contrast for adequate imaging. In addition, it is only possible to scan a selected area of the spine with this technique, and therefore one has to know the level of the pathology accurately to allow it to be imaged. Random slices taken by CT at various spinal levels are very likely to miss the true pathology. A further possible source of error exists if there is obvious bony pathology on plain X-rays such as a wedged vetebra. This may direct CT attention to this level when a myelogram will on many occasions show that the responsible pathology exists at a totally different level with the wedged vertebra being merely coincidental.

## SPINAL INJURY

Spinal injury is an excellent example of a neurological problem in which the final outcome can be drastically affected by the quality of the immediate medical care given. It is extremely rare for a spinal injury to occur in circumstances where the initial medical attendant has particular expertise in this matter. Any medical practitioner may be called upon to give immediate care to such patients. If the spinal injury is promptly recognised and appropriately treated, the patient is given not only the optimum chance of recovery but also the minimum chance of being made neurologically worse. Nothing is more tragic than the patient who sustains a spinal injury which initially does not damage the cord but in whom inexpert management allows the cord to become damaged by injudicious movement of the patient.

Spinal injuries can be categorised in several ways but perhaps the most important differentiation is between an injury that damages the spinal column alone, sparing the neural tissue within, and one that produces neurological damage as well. In the latter case, it is also important to decide whether the cord damage is complete or incomplete with partial sparing of some tracts, and also whether the lesion is permanent or whether recovery is likely. A major part of the processes that allow such decisions to be made depends on an accurate account of the initial situation and any subsequent change.

The diagnosis of a spinal injury can be totally straightforward or extremely difficult, demanding a high rate of suspicion. On the one hand, a conscious patient may be able to give an account of severe pain in the spine with altered sensation and lack of movement which makes the diagnosis obvious; whereas, on the other hand, the diagnosis may be extremely difficult in an unconscious patient. In such cases one has to look for clues indicating the presence of spinal injury. Indirect clues may be present such as the mechanism of the accident. High-velocity motor accidents, falls from a height and diving injuries are potent sources of spinal injury whereas such injuries are more unusual following, say, a direct blow to the head. The presence of lacerations on the forehead or occiput may indicate, respectively, an extension of flexion injury to the cervical spine.

The first stage of the assessment of these patients is to follow the rules of all trauma and to ensure that a patent airway is present and that there is no life-threatening haemorrhage. The maintenance of a patent airway in a patient with an injury to the cervical spine is not easy. Although several authorities suggest that the semi-prone position should be used to help airway potency, placing the spinally injured into this position may compromise the spine. It is best to leave the patient in the position in which he is found and to rely on an oral airway to protect respiration.

Upon the suspicion of injury to the spine it is necessary to examine the spine carefully, looking for any obvious deformity. Such examination in itself requires to be performed carefully. In the cervical spine, deformity may be obvious from the position in which the neck and head are lying. Lower in the spine, however, deformity will only be seen when the spine is examined. This requires the patient to be carefully 'log rolled' by at least three people rotating the patient in one piece to prevent any unwanted spinal movement. Injury may be apparent by the appearance of an obvious deformity or gibbus, but more usually less obvious signs are present such as widening of an interspinous gap, local tenderness or bruising.

The next crucial stage is the performance of an initial brief but thorough neurological examination. Assuming all else to be under control, it is best if this can be performed at the earliest opportunity, ideally at the scene of the accident. This is an important examination as it gives a baseline from which any further changes for better or worse can be gauged. In the conscious patient, the examination follows the methods already outlined in this chapter, with particular attention being paid to the presence and level of any sensory change or motor disturbance. It is particularly important to assess accurately the upper level of the neurological deficit as subsequent change in this is a vital factor. This demands knowledge of both sensory dermatomes and motor innervation of muscles. In broad terms, the dermatomes in the upper limb start with C5 on the lateral part of the upper arm and progress down the radial aspect until the middle finger is reached where the innervation is C8. From there they ascend up the ulnar border into the axilla where the innervation is T2. In the lower limb, dermatomes tend to wrap round the limb from lateral to medial, starting with L1 at the anterior iliac spine and passing down to S1 at the lateral border of the foot. Motor innervation is more difficult to remember, but guidelines may be taken from the following: shoulder abduction is mainly C5; elbow flexion is C5/6; wrist dorsiflexion is C7; and the small muscles of the hand are T1. In the lower limb, hip flexion is L1/2; knee extension is L3/4; ankle dorsiflexion is L5; and the hamstrings are mainly S1/2. Not too much importance needs to be placed on other factors such as tendon reflexes, plantars, etc., as often at this stage in the presence of cord injury spinal shock will be present which will abolish such signs completely. Even in the presence of an apparently severe neurological deficit, it is important to search for the presence of any voluntary function distal to the level of the cord lesion. The presence of even minor sensation or movement in the toes indicates that, although very severe, the lesion is incomplete; a situation with a much better prognosis than if it were complete.

In the unconscious patient, neurological assessment is much more difficult. One has to rely on the presence or absence of facial grimacing to deep painful stimuli such as pressing hard with a pen in the nail beds of fingers and toes to assess sensory function. Motor function can only be observed. For example an unconscious patient who is perhaps thrashing his arms about but in whom no movement in the legs is seen has to be assumed to have a spinal injury at some level below the neck. Somewhat more difficult is the cervically injured patient who shows no motor response. If such a patient is, for example, able to open his eyes and is perhaps giving some verbal response to examination, then that level of consciousness is at variance with the profound motor deficit and a cervical injury should be assumed.

One area of specific importance to the assessment of prognosis in spinal injury is the examination of sacral reflexes. Injury to the spinal cord is usually associated with the development of spinal shock. The phase of spinal shock is usually complete within the first 48 hours but it can persist from a few hours to several weeks. Spinal shock represents the phase during which no electrical activity is present in the isolated cord segment distal to the lesion. Gradually, as the intrinsic reflex function of the isolated segment returns, there is a return of the purely cord-mediated reflexes which persist in the functionally separate caudal segments. The presence or absence of such reflexes is of crucial importance to the ultimate prognosis of return of cord function as, if sacral reflexes have reappeared having been absent, it indicates that spinal shock has disappeared. If such a situation pertains with returned sacral reflexes in the absence of any return of voluntary mediated function distal to the level of a complete cord injury, most authorities would agree that there will be no recovery of voluntary function.

The main sacral reflexes referred to above are described below. The bulbocavernosus reflex is an appreciable contraction of the anus felt by a finger inserted rectally in response to gentle squeezing of the glans penis. The anal reflex is more easily elicited in the acute stage, being a visible anal contraction in response to a perianal pin-prick. The so-called malignant Strumpell reflex is a prolonged extensor response of the great toe following Babinski's manoeuvre. Finally, the presence of priapism in the early stages of a cord injury is a poor prognostic sign.

Although the examination of the patient has been discussed in a fair amount of detail, it should take only a few minutes to complete at the scene of the accident or at the first point of contact with a medical practitioner. Having completed this and attended to the airway and any associated major injuries, it is necessary to transport the patient to an appropriate place for further treatment to continue. Even if the diagnosis of spinal injury is only suspected at this stage, it is necessary to take the greatest care when transporting such patients. It is perhaps obvious to state that this is also true of the situation of a patient suspected of having a spinal injury but who has no evidence of neurological damage at the time, as injudicious movement of such a patient may be very dangerous if an unstable spinal column injury has occurred.

In certain circumstances it is necessary to move a patient prior to performing the assessment outlined above as, for example, in a patient trapped in a vehicle following a road traffic accident. In that situation it should always be assumed that spinal injury has occurred and the patient has to be extricated with great care, moving him in 'one piece' with reference to the spine. This often requires the services of several people to maintain spinal alignment. Several ambulances carry special boards such as a Hines cervical splint which can be inserted *in situ* to allow safer removal. However, it has to be stressed that less secure pieces of apparatus such as conventional cervical collars or the oft suggested rolled-up newspaper afford no protection to the spine and are dangerous as they only instil a false sense of security.

Having assessed the patient, it is necessary to transfer him or her on to a stretcher for further transportation. The best method available is the 'scoop' type of spinal stretcher which can be gently inserted under the patient from each side. If such a stretcher is not available, then the patient must be lifted in one piece, an action requiring at least three people to take the trunk and limbs and with an additional attendant responsible for the neck and head. Again it has to be stated that the patient is not safe even when on the stretcher, and requires continuing physical support during transfer. Unless there are associated life-threatening injuries, the transfer to hospital should not be made at high speed as a more sedate pace is less likely to be injurious. One further aspect of transfer is worthy of note. Patients with a high cervical cord injury lose vasomotor control and as a consequence may quickly become relatively hypothermic and hypotensive. The former is easy to prevent by use of appropriate blankets or 'space blankets' if available. The latter can, however, prompt medical attendants into rapid volume transfusion, which can be very dangerous.

On arrival at hospital, the general and neurological examination has to be repeated, and appropriate essential general measures must be undertaken. Once stabilised, high-quality radiographs of the injured area of the spine are required, a practice which requires considerable radiographic skills. Obvious fractures should be easily diagnosed, but some can be very difficult to image. Such difficult examples include: the cervico-thoracic fracture which is easily obscured by the shoulders; the high cervical fracture of C1 or C2 and fractures in children. It must be appreciated that not all spinal injuries produce fractures and/or misalignment. Pure dislocations, though rare, do occur as do pure disc injuries which may show no abnormality at all on a plain radiograph. In some cases misalignment which occurred at the time of injury may have spontaneously reduced, restoring normal alignment. In such cases the only radiographic clue may be the presence of soft tissue swelling, indicating a prevertebral haematoma or a minor increase in the interspinous distance indicating soft tissue damage.

Having established the diagnosis of spinal injury the next important action is to restore spinal alignment as quickly and atraumatically as possible. This is necessary in order to restore the cross-sectional area of the spinal canal to as near as normal as possible so as to relieve any mechanical compression of the spinal cord. There are basically three methods which can be employed: gradual controlled reduction with traction; acute manipulative reduction; and operative reduction. The most commonly employed method is the first. However, even this technique requires considerable skill. In outline, with reference to a cervical fracture, skull traction is employed by the insertion of one of the various types of skull caliper, perhaps the most common being those of Gardner's design. The insertion of these is quite critical in that, if they are inserted at the incorrect place in the skull and with the incorrect degree of tension, not only is intracranial haemorrhage or infection a possibility but also the incorrect insertion will lead to an improperly aligned traction pull which may interfere with reduction. The patient should then, if there are no contraindications, be given some combination of sedation and muscle relaxant to counteract the effects of the muscle spasm associated with such injuries, and traction weights are then applied. The direction of the traction pull at this stage is quite critical and depends on the mechanism of injury. For example, in a case of a flexion–rotation injury leading perhaps to a bilateral facet dislocation with anterior subluxation of the superior vertebral body on the inferior, the initial pull has to produce more flexion in order to disengage the locked facets. Weights up to 20 kg (45 lb) may be necessary in a well built man to produce this result, but the traction should be added slowly and incrementally to that level with frequent radiographs or screening being taken to follow the progress of reduction. Once the facets are disengaged it is necessary to change the direction of traction into extension to complete reduction, and then to reduce the weight to the order of 7–9 kg (15–20 lb) to maintain the reduction. A major word of caution is necessary with regard to the traction weight used in fractures of the upper cervical spine as the normal countering muscle pull at that level is much decreased and the use of greater than 4.5 kg (10 lb) may cause serious overdistraction.

The use of acute manipulative reduction must only be applied by experienced operators as it is potentially a much more hazardous technique than the gradual method outlined above. Here, the patient is cautiously anaesthetised and under X-ray screening the manoeuvres described already are conducted smoothly but quickly to effect reduction. Particularly if there is only a unilateral facet dislocation, it is also necessary to rotate the neck in the correct direction. This manoeuvre, correctly performed, does allow the quickest spinal realignment and reduction. Following reduction by either method, it is necessary to continue with skull traction to immobilise the spine and prevent redislocation. Even though the patient is maintained in traction, it is a fallacy to believe that he is now safe, and skilled nursing on special turning frames or electric beds is necessary to prevent dislocation.

Only if either of the above methods fails should operative reduction be considered necessary, a highly complicated procedure requiring an additional fusion at the same time. The only exception to the above rules about spinal realignment comes in the instance of a delayed diagnosis where the fracture–dislocation is not recognised in the first two weeks following injury. Reduction by any method is highly dangerous at that stage, and the fracture position normally has to be accepted.

For years there has been debate about the role of urgent surgery and other therapies such as steroids, barbiturates and local spinal cord cooling in the treatment of spinal injury with neurological deficit. It is fair to say that as yet none of the methods suggested has been shown with certainty to improve the neurological outcome in such patients. The biggest debate has been regarding the role of acute surgery. There are several papers claiming successful neurological outcome following major interventional surgery. The problem is, of course, that a significant number of patients improve neurologically following the conservative therapy outlined above, and it is true to say that no controlled study has shown that a surgically treated group fares better neurologically than a conservative group. The three facts that are clear about surgery, however, are that: first, laminectomy alone is not only useless but also compromises further the spinal stability; secondly, if surgery is considered, it must be performed by an experienced spinal surgeon; and, finally, the only situation where surgery is obligatory is in the relatively rare occurrence of increasing neurological deficit following injury, reinforcing the need for an accurate early baseline neurological examination. The role of surgery in the later stages of management in order to fuse the spine and allow earlier mobilisation is beyond the scope of this book.

**FURTHER READING**

Edmondson, A.S. and Cranshaw, A.H. (eds) (1980) *Campbell's operative orthopaedics* 6th edn, C.V. Mosby, St. Louis, Mo.

Northfield, D.C. (in press) *Surgery of the central nervous system*, 2nd edn, Blackwell Scientific Publications, Oxford

Rothman, R.H. and Simeone, F.A. (1982) *The spine*, W.B. Saunders, Philadelphia

# 12

# Pain as a Neurological Emergency

David Bowsher

## INTRODUCTION

Pain has been officially defined (by the International Association for the Study of Pain, IASP) as 'an unpleasant physical and emotional experience, due to tissue damage or described in terms of such'. Like other sensations, pain has a *perception threshold*; and, like other sensations, its threshold is relatively constant (about 45°C). What varies from person to person, and even in the same individual at different times, is *pain tolerance*, defined as *the greatest degree of pain a subject is able to tolerate*. It is most important to realise that patients do not seek medical advice about pain until they have gone *beyond the tolerance level*, and the pain has become *in*tolerable.

Pain is the commonest reason for seeking medical advice, and is said to be the presenting symptom in about one-third of all consultations. Frequently it is an indicator, useful to the doctor if not to the patient, of underlying pathology the treatment of which will successfully abolish the pain. A number of conditions, however, result in *intractable chronic pain*; these include not only malignant disease, in which there is (generally unjustified) fear of dying in pain, but also such diseases as osteoarthritis, as well as the neurogenic pains to be discussed below, in all of which the patient may be condemned for many years to live in pain. In recent years, a large number of specialist pain-relief clinics have come into existence; if intractable pain cannot be quickly and successfully relieved in primary care, patients should be referred to such clinics sooner rather than later.

Two types of pain, either of which can present as an emergency, fall within the ambit of neurology. These are headache and neurogenic pain (see below). However, since all pain is a result of activity within the nervous system, a final section of this chapter will be devoted to the treatment of other forms of chronic pain.


## HEADACHE

Careful and accurate history taking is the key to virtually all neurological diagnosis, and nowhere is this more true than in the differential diagnosis of headache. Perhaps the simplest approach is to make a checklist of questions, such as:

(a) Where in/on the head is it?
(b) How long have you had it? Is it getting worse, better, or staying the same?
(c) Is it continuous or throbbing? (This question is of little diagnostic value to the physician, but patients expect to be asked it! And it may help to lead into the more useful question: Can you describe what it *feels* like?, which if put without preliminaries too frequently elicits unhelpful replies such as 'Awful'.)
(d) Have you had a headache like this before? If so, when did it first occur? What is the frequency and duration of attacks?
(e) Are you taking any drugs (NB: non-steroidal anti-inflammatory drugs (NSAIDs)), and particularly, have you recently started on a new drug? Have you eaten or drunk anything unusual, or to your knowledge been exposed to any unusual chemical in the environment?
(f) What do you [the patient] think may be causing your headache?
(g) Are there any concomitant symptoms/signs? (Hypertension, nausea, vomiting, faintness or more serious alterations of consciousness, photophobia, sweating, pains elsewhere, constipation or diarrhoea, fever, pupillary change, drug inges-tion, etc.: hypertensive headache, usually worst on waking (because recumbent BP is higher than upright BP), is said to be rare with diastolic pressures below 110 mmHg.)

Headache may of course be the presenting symptom of many febrile exanthemata or infections (do not forget meningitis!), or of intestinal, hepatic, or renal insufficiencies, none of which is within the domain of the present chapter. Neurosurgical headaches have been dealt with in Chapter 10, but it is worth reiterating the fact that the sudden blinding headache which nearly always denotes the onset of subarachnoid or cerebral haemorrhage, apart from its (usual) severity, is more remarkable for being described as being 'like nothing I ever felt before'. Neck stiffness occurs in meningitis and subarachnoid haemorrhage, but not usually in cerebral haemorrhage.

Space-occupying intracranial lesions are usually, but not always, accompanied by headache. Such headaches tend to be generalised unless the pathological process involves the meninges at a specific point. Drowsiness and papilloedema may clinch the diagnosis. Always remember that personality change in middle age *without* headache may be due to a frontal lobe tumour; perform an ophthalmoscopic examination or even get a neurological/neurosurgical opinion before deciding that the case is definitely psychiatric.

'Essential' headaches are usually divided into vascular and muscle contraction types. Vascular headaches are represented by classical migraine, cluster headache and cranial arteritis. There is rarely much difficulty in diagnosing the typical sick headache of classical migraine, even though it may not be a hemicrania (but it usually starts on one side before spreading): there may have been a visual or gastric aura; there is often a family history; and of course there is usually a history of previous attacks. Failure to respond to the 'usual' treatment within a few hours is the usual reason for which migraine may present as an emergency. If ergotamine has not already been used, it should be administered intramuscularly (0.5 mg ergotamine tartrate) immediately the diagnosis has been made. If there is no improvement in 30 minutes, 2 mg of the drug may be taken sublingually — and repeated up to a total dose of 6 mg. This will take 1½ hours; if there is no improvement by 2 hours, other means will have to be used. Buclizine hydrochloride 13 mg is effective in some cases, but any remedy that has not been tried previously should be used. If no relief is obtained by specific treatment (which may include feverfew or acupuncture), there is nothing to do but leave the patient in a darkened room with analgesics such as paracetamol and the assurance that the headache *will* get better. If it persists for 72 hours, it is wise to consider another diagnosis, and to begin investigation in an attempt to establish the cause.

Cluster headache ('migrainous neuralgia') is so called because the headaches tend to be clustered in time. It is more likely than classical migraine to result in an emergency call, because the pain strikes suddenly, often in the middle of the night. The pain is always unilateral, frequently centred on the orbit ('behind the eye'), often accompanied by conjunctival injection and/or lacrimation and/or rhinorrhoea. The pain is usually described as boring or burning, and is commoner in men than in women; unlike migraine, it frequently does not begin until middle age. Each attack rarely lasts more than an hour, but may be so severe as to cause the patient to consider suicide. Once an attack starts, it is likely to be followed by a 'cluster' of attacks, which can come up to a dozen (but more frequently three or four) times a day and last for weeks. During an attack, there is tenderness on pressure over the branches of the common and external carotid arteries. Abortive treatment is with ergotamine, as for classical migraine. In some refractory cases, good results have been reported with steroids (prednisone, up to 80 mg per day).

Cranial arteritis causes a persistent throbbing pain, usually in the temporal region; if the pain spreads, it is more likely to go down into the face than up to the vertex. The giveaway diagnostic feature is the exquisite tenderness of the (often distended) branches of the external carotid artery — usually the temporal artery. The condition may be due to generalised arterial disease (polyarteritis nodosa) or to localised pure cranial arteritis. The great danger is to vision; photophobia and even diplopia occur in a substantial proportion of cases. Immediate treatment with steroids should be instituted as soon as the diagnosis is made.

Muscle contraction headache, usually known as tension headache, is most often described as a tight band around the head, or a 'vice-like' pain. It is frequently occipital, sometimes fronto-occipital; it is very rare for it to be unilateral. Women are more frequently afflicted than men. Since the headache is very often associated with (caused by, according to some) anxiety, it is not uncommon for medical aid to be sought as an emergency. Again, history is all-important in helping establish the diagnosis. Tender spots can nearly always be found in the nuchal and/or occipito-frontal muscles. If there is any limitation of neck movements, or if neck movements cause pain, cervical spondylosis or cervical osteoarthritis should be suspected as a cause. Injection of tender spots with local anaesthetic may relieve the pain 'miraculously'. In addition to analgesics such as paracetamol, diazepam is helpful because it is a muscle relaxant as well as being an anxiolytic.

## NEUROGENIC PAIN

Most pain is caused by the excitation of specific *nociceptor nerve endings* in skin or deep tissues. The majority of headaches, for instance, arise from the excitation of such nerve endings in the meninges, generally the dura mater, or their contained blood vessels. Some nociceptors, particularly in the skin, are specifically activated by high-threshold mechanical or thermal stimuli, but most (in deep tissues as well as skin) are phylogenetically ancient chemoreceptors connected to unmyelinated (C) nerve fibres. They are known as *polymodal nociceptors*, because they are apparently activated by mechanical, thermal or chemical stimuli. The real reason for this is believed to be that the true activator is a chemical substance which is liberated, or comes into being, as a result of tissue damage — whether that damage be provoked by mechanical, thermal or chemical (e.g. inflammation) means. This, of course, is why pain sensation usually outlasts the apparently provoking stimulus.

Neurogenic pain, on the other hand, *does not arise as the result of nerve terminal excitation, but because of damage to axons in the peripheral or central nervous system.* We are thus talking about painful conditions such as post-herpetic and trigeminal neuralgia, causalgia, and so-called 'thalamic syndrome', to name but a few. Taken together, neurogenic pains are common; they account for more than 25% of all patients seen at the very large (> 3000 patients per year) pain-relieving clinic at Walton Hospital in Liverpool. The incidence of neurogenic pain increases with age, so that it accounts for one-third of all patients over the age of 65, and one-half of those over 70. In an ageing population, therefore, neurogenic pain must be taken very seriously.

Although the causes of neurogenic pain are legion, its manifestations and its treatment are fairly uniform. Thus, despite the woefully inadequate state of knowledge about its pathophysiology, it does seem to be more or less an entity, albeit with a number of recognisable subcategories. Its main distinguishing features are:

(1) Patients frequently complain of a *shooting* and/or *burning* pain, often in addition to more familiar descriptions such as aching or throbbing.

(2) *Neurogenic pain does not respond to narcotic analgesics.* Large doses of analgesics may 'take the edge off the pain' in some cases, but there is no real analgesic effect. Although the failure

of narcotics to relieve neurogenic pain is virtually pathognomonic of neurogenic pain, it is hardly recommended as a method of diagnosis! It is better *not* to use them, having made a correct diagnosis by other means. Pain-relieving clinics have to detoxify far too many geriatric junkies before rational treatment of neurogenic pain can be initiated.

(3) With the notable exception of trigeminal neuralgia (and the very rare glossopharyngeal neuralgia), neurogenic pain is always accompanied by a neurological deficit. There is a tendency (and no more than a tendency) for the deficit in *peripheral* neurogenic pains to be of those somatosensory submodalities normally carried by large primary afferent fibres — touch, vibration, etc.; whereas in central conditions the deficit may involve those submodalities, such as temperature and pin-prick, normally carried by small peripheral fibres.

(4) There is frequently an autonomic dysfunction, most typically seen perhaps in the 'trophic' skin changes of causalgia, when the skin is red, shiny and hot. Sweating is frequently affected, in either direction, so that the skin is either dryer or wetter than the corresponding area on the other side. Skin temperature too is frequently altered; contact thermography suggests that it is virtually always cooler than the contralateral unaffected area. This last is the only objective autonomic change apparently found in trigeminal neuralgia (see below). But the feature that most frequently emerges on questioning, or sometimes even spontaneously, is that the pain is aggravated by emotional events such as being angry or upset, and also by orgasm; and sometimes partly alleviated by rest, relaxation, and emotional calmness.

(5) The sleep pattern is rarely disturbed by neurogenic pains, despite their severity. This can sometimes be difficult to elicit, because these usually elderly patients often say that they have difficulty in getting off to sleep, or can't do so without a hypnotic. However, careful questioning will usually show that this was the case before the onset of the painful condition. These patients usually have no more difficulty in getting off to sleep than before the onset of the neurogenic pain, though they may wake in agony.

(6) *Allodynia* — the elicitation of pain by a normally non-painful stimulus — is a common feature of neurogenic pain. A good example is the trigger points of trigeminal neuralgia, when a stimulus such as the presence of food in the mouth or of the wind

on the cheek may set off the pain. In a number of other conditions, rubbing may be the most effective stimulus: it is not uncommon to see post-herpetic patients who go to the most elaborate lengths to prevent their clothes from rubbing their skin. Yet firm grasping of, for example, an allodynic limb in causalgia or thalamic syndrome may not be pain-provoking, or may even relieve the pain for a moment or two. Cold allodynia is particularly common in neurogenic pains. This may be revealed by the patient's report that 'My pain is worse when it's cold' — but can easily be elicited by a cold stimulus, such as an ice cube applied to the skin.

(7) Irradiation of pain is also commonly seen: elicited pain spreads out from the point at which it was originally provoked.

Guided by the presence of these characteristic features, it should not be difficult to know when a pain is neurogenic; so it is hoped that it will rarely prove necessary to clinch the point by the time-consuming exercise of demonstrating that the pain does not respond to analgesics — for this, if persisted in, can also damage the patient and make true relief harder to achieve. The actual type of neurogenic pain concerned can be diagnosed by a consideration of the history and the distribution of the pain.

Neurogenic pains characterised *only* by shooting pain, and not by burning, stand in a class of their own, and should be dealt with separately. The type-example of this is of course trigeminal neuralgia, which will be described here, together with its treatment; other types of 'pure' shooting pain will then be considered.

### Trigeminal neuralgia

In its idiopathic form, trigeminal neuralgia is most commonly first seen from the seventh decade onwards. However, it has been observed in children, and a first attack has been reported by a subject over 100 years old. The second or third division (*not* the first) is the usual site of pain; and it is slightly commoner on the right side than the left.

The first attack (like many subsequent ones) comes out of the blue. It is described as a stabbing, shooting, jabbing, lancinating, pain, 'like an electric shock' in the face, lasting only a few seconds. As the attack is so short and the pain goes away, often not to reappear for some time, it is very rare for patients to seek medical advice after the first attack, though it should be stressed that severity (as opposed to frequency) may be maximal from the first. Further attacks occur, and their frequency increases, causing the patient to consult a doctor (or dentist). In the advanced case, where the patient does not wash or shave the affected side of the face and can describe a trigger zone, diagnosis is of course very easy. But what this book is about is early diagnosis and treatment. What does one do in the case of a patient who reports a few brief attacks of stabbing pain, which do not occur during the consultation?

(a) Test sensation on both sides of the face with cotton wool and a pin; no change will be observed in cases of true idiopathic trigeminal neuralgia.
(b) Try to set off the pain by finding a trigger zone on the face, on the inner side of the cheek, on the teeth or gums, or even on the tongue.

This form of physical examination will afford the opportunity of excluding dental or gingival disease; pressing over the paranasal (particularly maxillary) sinuses will help to exclude sinusitis. More difficult to exclude is a form of masticatory dysfunction syndrome, sometimes known as temporo-mandibular joint (TMJ) dysfunction. Stabbing pains occur about 1 cm in front of the joint; they are usually associated with jaw movement, not necessarily mastication. The pains do not occur every time the jaw is moved, so may not be provoked by the examiner. However, the stabbing pain is *never* truly spontaneous. In addition to the stabbing pains, a dull ache, sometimes persisting all day, is characteristic of all forms of masticatory dysfunction syndrome. The patient will frequently have a mechanical jaw closure problem, perhaps associated with misaligned dentures or gingival shrinkage with age. Those given to nocturnal tooth grinding (audible) or jaw clenching (silent) are also prone to develop the condition. Geniculate herpes zoster (see below) can also cause diagnostic problems.

If the above can be excluded, the possibilities of cluster headache and 'atypical facial pain' remain; the latter can be very difficult on purely clinical grounds. However, a recent investigation in our Department with contact thermography (P.A.J. Hardy, personal communication) has shown in fifteen successive cases of idiopathic trigeminal neuralgia that the affected side of the face is cooler than the normal, whereas in atypical facial pain it is either warmer (as it is, of course, in all infections and inflammations) or isothermic.

If thermography is unavailable, a sensitive skin thermometer may be used; otherwise diagnosis must be made by the unaided acumen of the physician. It may be helpful to take the patient's age into consideration; the younger the patient, the more unlikely (though not impossible) is true trigeminal neuralgia. So long as possibly serious organic disease can be ruled out, therapeutic trial with carbamazepine may be undertaken, since the drug is virtually specific: 100 mg should be taken at night for the first 3 days, then 100 mg night and morning; after the first week, the dose can be increased to 100 mg three times a day, and should be held at this level for 2 weeks. If the effect is insufficient, the dose can be increased by 100 mg a week up to a daily maximum of 800 mg. It may eventually be necessary (see below) to increase dosage up to 1200 mg/day. But at higher levels plasma concentration should be monitored; optimal levels are between 13 and a maximum of 42 micromoles/litre (3–10 microgrammes/ml).

(1) Carbamazepine is not an analgesic, so no effect will be seen on taking the first few doses; indeed it is not usual to see any effect for about a week. It is *most important* to make sure the patient understands this — not only in the case of trigeminal neuralgia, but all other neurogenic pains as well (see below). Far too many patients try a drug for a few days and the give it up, saying 'It didn't take the pain away, Doctor', unless they are warned. They must also be warned about the possible side effects of the drug (particularly dizziness and drowsiness, less frequently gastro-intestinal disturbances; if a rash develops, they must *stop* taking the drug); and they must be assured that these effects are likely to pass off after the first few days.

(2) How long should the therapeutic trial last? If no effect whatsoever is obtained after one month, the trial may be abandoned and the patient sent for specialist investigation and advice, with reasonable certainty that, whatever the condition is, it is *not* trigeminal neuralgia. More often, though, the patient may report some slight improvement after a fortnight or even a month. Provided that one can be sure that this is not being said to 'please the doctor' (and because the patient has faith in the doctor, and *believes* that the doctor must be making him/her better), i.e. is a placebo effect, then the dose can be gradually and cautiously increased until relief is obtained.

(3) Although virtually self-evident, it should perhaps be stated that there is no point in carrying out a therapeutic trial until the

attacks are sufficiently frequent to allow one to be certain after a couple of weeks that drugs *are* having an effect. By rule of thumb, this means an attack every two days or at the very least twice a week. In fact, patients do not often seek advice until this sort of frequency is attained.

It is not recognised that many cases of trigeminal neuralgia are not 'idiopathic', but symptomatic of, for example, an aberrant blood vessel, a fibrous band, or even a tumour. For this reason, more active treatment is frequently undertaken; for example, some neurosurgeons perform posterior fossa craniotomy on all otherwise healthy cases under the age of 60. Among the conditions that are now thought to be causative may be mentioned aberrant intracranial blood vessels. Multiple sclerosis is a cause *not* calling for surgical intervention, but may be picked up if:

(a) the patient is relatively young, and/or
(b) there is a sensory deficit in the face, and/or
(c) there is a history of visual disturbance, and/or
(d) there are changes in the optic disc on ophthalmoscopic examination, or
(e) there are any other manifestations of multiple sclerosis.

In any event, the majority of cases of trigeminal neuralgia eventually escape from control by carbamazepine, even though the dose may have been increased up to about 800 mg/day in divided doses. Other anticonvulsants — sodium valproate (valproic acid), phenytoin — may be tried, but invasive methods are usually necessary at this stage. The method of choice is most frequently percutaneous radiofrequency differential thermocoagulation; but both cryosurgery and glycerol injection, both effected percutaneously, are popular in some clinics. All these methods ideally spare the ophthalmic division of the nerve entirely, and also (though with less certainty) low-threshold mechanoreceptive function in the affected divisions(s).

It was as long ago as 1885 that Trousseau described trigeminal neuralgia as a form of 'sensory epilepsy'; and this was the rationale for its treatment by anticonvulsants, though none was really satisfactory until the advent of carbamazepine in 1962. At the present time it may seem more practical to stand this axiom on its head and say that shooting neurogenic pains can usually be treated with anticonvulsants. This applies not only to the neuralgias currently under discussion, but also to the shooting element of the symptomatically mixed

225

neurogenic pains to be described in the next section of this chapter.

Metatarsalgia is generally recognised as a true (but rare) neuralgic shooting pain occurring in the distribution indicated by its name, and should be treated with anticonvulsants. Another form of shooting pain which may present as an emergency is the lightning pain of *tabes dorsalis*. The history will usually establish the diagnosis. It is perhaps more obvious with tabes than with some other neuralgias that the pain is exacerbated (i.e. the attacks are more frequent) at times of emotional stress. This is in accordance with the general rules of neurogenic pain, and shows that even neuralgias may have an autonomic component. In our experience, the drug of first choice in tabes is sodium valproate (valproic acid), in an initial dose of 200 mg at night, increasing after 1 week to 200 mg morning and evening, and after a further week to 200 mg three times a day after food. It is rarely necessary to go to doses higher than 600 or 800 mg/day for the control of shooting pain (in tabes dorsalis or any other condition), although for epilepsy daily doses as high as 2400 mg are used. The optimal plasma concentration is said to be from 278 to 694 micromoles per litre, and the lower part of this range is likely to be effective for shooting pains. The drug is occasionally hepatotoxic, especially during the first few months of administration, so both clinical (vomiting, jaundice, anorexia, weakness) and serological signs of liver failure should be carefully looked for. For patients on long-term treatment with sodium valproate, many clinicians consider it prudent to carry out liver function tests every three to six months. Heartburn is a common side effect at the beginning of treatment, about which the patient must be warned. Over the longer term, weight gain is not infrequent.

Any form of nerve compression can cause shooting pains. Thus it can occur in cancer, due to entrapment of a nerve in the tumour mass, or more frequently to compression due to vertebral collapse, resulting in girdle or hemigirdle pains. Vertebral collapse of course frequently occurs suddenly in cancer, giving rise to a sudden access of shooting pain for which the physician will be called. Such patients are frequently already under treatment by narcotics; but anticonvulsants should now be added.

Two forms of curable nerve compression give rise to shooting pains. One is prolapsed intervertebral disc (PID), giving rise to sciatica in the lower limb; the other is carpal tunnel syndrome, affecting the upper limb. If surgery has to be deferred, or for some reason cannot be performed, the exhibition of anticonvulsants can have a pain-relieving effect.

Neurogenic pains characterised by shooting *and* burning, together with or without other types of pain such as throbbing, aching or squeezing (compression), or burning alone, with or without any other types of pain, form another category, to be differentiated from the pure shooting pains. There is, unfortunately, no generic name for this category of painful conditions, but they may be considered as *peripheral* or *central* neurogenic pains — it being understood that the pure shooting neuralgias are excluded. These conditions are all clinically very similar, and are mainly differentiated on the basis of history and distribution of pain.

Neurogenic pains of this type can occur in a number of systemic diseases, of which the commonest is probably painful diabetic neuropathy; vitamin B12 deficiency is another example. General neurogenic pain of this type should of course disappear as the underlying condition is treated; but it may prove intractable, particularly in the case of diabetic neuropathy. If it is necessary to treat these pains symptomatically, they should be treated in the same way as, for example, post-herpetic neuralgia (see below), and *not* with conventional analgesics.

**Peripheral neurogenic pains**

By far the commonest form of neurogenic pain is of course *post-herpetic neuralgia*, which is said to follow one-tenth of all cases of herpes zoster (itself by far the commonest disease affecting the nervous system), but more like 50% of those occurring in patients over 70 years of age. It usually follows directly on from shingles without a break, but there may be a pain-free interval between the attack of acute zoster and the onset of painful post-herpetic neuralgia. Post-herpetic neuralgia is in fact defined as pain present one month after the rash has healed. Somewhat over half of all cases of shingles occur in thoracic dermatomes (particularly T5), and another quarter in the ophthalmic division of the trigeminal nerve.

The diagnosis of post-herpetic neuralgia is usually perfectly obvious from the history, scars of the rash, distribution and description of the pain. However, it may occasionally present as an emergency in cases where the rash was minimal, or completely healed; or where it cannot be seen (the classical example is geniculate herpes, characterised by the onset of pain which is shooting in nature) and so cause confusion with trigeminal neuralgia; careful examination of the external auditory meatus (including comparison with that on the other side) will usually reveal a vesicular rash or its cicatrices.

Although the pain of post-herpetic neuralgia is typically described as burning and/or shooting, in our experience a large number of patients complain of aching, dragging or 'boring' pains. The painful area may be exquisitely tender (allodynic), and patients will sometimes go to extraordinary lengths to prevent clothes moving across the affected region of skin,binding themselves into veritable cuirasses of unmovable material.

The first duty of the attending physician is to do all within his or her power to try to stop post-herpetic neuralgia from developing. This means taking acute herpes zoster very seriously indeed; it must *never* be dismissed as just another irritating plague of the elderly, to be treated with sedatives, mild analgesics, and placebo. This said, it must immediately be admitted that there *is* no satisfactory treatment of acute shingles that will guarantee the prevention of the development of post-herpetic neuralgia. However, vigorous treatment of an erupted rash with idoxuridine or topical acyclovir should always be carried out. Antiviral treatment with systemic acyclovir (4 g/day, in divided doses, for 7 days) is also recommended. Immediate sympathetic blockade (where this is practicable — i.e. stellate ganglion block for ophthalmic herpes) is advocated by some. Claims have also been made for the immediate institution, as soon as the diagnosis is made, of small nocturnal doses of a tricyclic antidepressant (e.g. amitriptyline 10 or 25 mg nocte); this should be kept up for a month or two. This therapy is cheap and easy, so there would appear to be little harm in recommending that it always be tried, in addition to other measures.

The treatment of post-herpetic neuralgia is that of all neurogenic pains characterised by burning as well as by shooting sensations. The most useful combination of drugs is that of a tricyclic and an anticonvulsant. Tricyclics (and bicyclics, but not tetracyclics) inhibit the reuptake of the neurotransmitters noradrenaline and 5-hydroxytryptamine (serotonin), and so potentiate their action. Both these transmitters are released by descending systems of supraspinal origin whose terminals are concerned with the inhibition of nociceptive circuits in the spinal cord. Since serotonin has been implicated in the activation of endogenous opioid mechanisms, and neurogenic pain is notoriously resistant to opiates, it may be that direct inhibition by noradrenergic neurones is more likely to be responsible for the therapeutic effect of tricyclics. Like anticonvulsants, the pain-relieving effect of tricyclics is not immediate but usually takes some weeks to develop; the patient must be warned of this.

The commencing dose should be small: 25 mg at night for younger patients, 10 mg for the elderly. Taking care not to produce side effects, the dose should be gradually increased until the patient is taking about 75 mg a day in divided doses (50 mg for the elderly). If burning persists after a month, the dose may be cautiously increased to a maximum of 150 mg/day for younger patients — about 100 mg for the aged. Some authorities believe that phenothiazines potentiate the action of tricyclics, and so advocate the use of a proprietary preparation consisting of tablets containing 25 mg of amitriptyline and 2 mg of perphenazine. An anticholinesterase such as distigmine may be substituted for or taken in addition to, a tricyolic.

Our own anticonvulsant of first choice is sodium valproate. We start with 200 mg at night and increase gradually to 200 mg two or three times a day; it is rarely necessary to go above 800 mg a day to combat the shooting pains of post-herpetic neuralgia. If no relief is obtained after a month other anticonvulsants (carbamazepine, phenytoin) should be tried.

Some additional therapy may be called for in certain cases of post-herpetic neuralgia. Most patients find that a local anaesthetic aerosol spray is helpful, even though the duration of action is short. If the patient demands an analgesic (and they usually do!), dihydrocodeine occasionally 'takes the edge off' the pain. It is the only analgesic we would be prepared to use; if its use is to be prolonged, its constipating effects must be countered, particularly in the elderly, with a preparation such as danthron. Where anatomically feasible, sympathetic blockade is certainly helpful. Surgical treatment by dorsal root entry zone (DREZ) microlesions has proved helpful in particularly intractable cases; also, recently developed techniques for percutaneous differential thermocoagulation of dorsal root ganglia may hopefully be expected to be useful.

The extent to which dorsal root ganglia are affected by the infectious viral process differs from case to case. A rough idea may be gained by simple clinical sensory testing. If a sufficient proportion of large peripheral fibres are intact, as revealed by the patient's ability to feel the touch of cotton wool in the affected dermatome, then transcutaneous electrical nerve stimulation (TENS) may be useful in peripheral neurogenic pain, including post-herpetic neuralgia, since it works through the non-opioid inhibitory action of large mechanoreceptive peripheral fibres on small nociceptive axons. Acupuncture, on the other hand, which appears to work

229

through an endorphinergic mechanism, is reported not to be of any help in post-herpetic neuralgia, or any other narcotic-resistant neurogenic pain.

The importance of vigorously instituting suitable treatment at the earliest possible moment cannot be sufficiently emphasised. The longer the condition is allowed to continue, the more difficult it becomes to treat effectively. This is really why both herpes zoster and post-herpetic neuralgia (and indeed any other neurogenic pain) should be considered as neurological emergencies.

*Causalgia* is a classical form of peripheral neurogenic pain, usually affecting a single nerve, most frequently the median or ulnar and less often the femoral. The agonising, typically burning, pain follows injury, always partial, to the nerve. Although most cases are traumatic in origin, the impression is growing that there is an increasing incidence of iatrogenic cases, consequent upon ulnar nerve transposition or lumbar disc surgery. There is almost always an interval of time between nerve injury and the onset of causalgic pain. The name *causalgia minor* has recently been applied to those distal forms of the disease that follow trauma such as Colles' fracture and are more familiar under the name of reflex sympathetic dystrophy or Sudek's atrophy.

In addition to the spontaneous pain, allodynia is nearly always marked: the patient cannot bear to be touched in the affected area; there are trophic changes in the skin, including autonomic dysfunction. It has been reported that the subcutaneous injection of 1 microgram of adrenaline, totally without effect in normal skin, brings on severe causalgic pain when performed in an affected area, thus underlining the important role of the sympathetic nervous system in the generation of neurogenic pain. In reflex sympathetic dystrophy or causalgia minor, there is usually also osteolysis.

The medical treatment used for post-herpetic neuralgia may give some relief in causalgia, but sympatholysis is the treatment of choice. Since, unlike post-herpetic neuralgia, the condition usually afflicts limbs, such procedures are technically feasible. If only the distal part of a limb is affected, depletion of adrenergic nerve terminals can be effected by the intravenous injection of guanethidine distal to a tourniquet; it is frequently necessary to repeat this at short intervals over 2 or 3 weeks in order to achieve a permanent result. When the upper parts of limbs are involved, it will be necessary to undertake sympatholytic injection of stellate or lumbar ganglia. Good results have been reported from medical treatment with the systemic administration of phenoxybenzamine, 10 mg t.d.s., increasing to 80 mg/day, for not more than a month; but the treatment has to be undertaken in hospital because of the resultant hypotension. Along the same lines, some success has been obtained in causalgia minor by treatment with ketanserin, an $\alpha_1$ and $5-HT_2$ blocker.

Intermediate between peripheral and central neurogenic pain is *brachial plexus avulsion* (or indeed any other root avulsion), most often seen after motor-cycle accidents and other trauma. Whereas the motor deficit due to lower motor neurone damage becomes apparent immediately, the severe burning pain may not appear until a certain time has passed – perhaps even after the patient has been discharged from a traumatology service, so that the pain may present as an emergency occurring at home. The pain is often felt in parts of the limb entirely bereft of sensation, and so is akin to phantom limb pain following amputation. In other (more frequent) cases, the pain occurs in a part of the limb in which the sensory deficit is subtotal. The immediate treatment should be sympatholysis (stellate ganglion blockade) if possible, and medical treatment with tricyclics and anticonvulsants certainly. Neurosurgical microlesions placed in the dorsal root entry zone (DREZ) of the spinal cord are said by its proponents to be helpful, and have also been used in other forms of neurogenic pain such as post-herpetic neuralgia.

*Phantom limb pain* is more obviously central, and may be entirely neurogenic in which case it should be treated in the same way as avulsion. More frequently, it is a mixture of neurogenic (as defined here) and other pain, in which the burning features may be less evident. Thus there may be a neuroma requiring injection or excision. Where peripheral nerve stimulation is practicable, it may be helpful. More often, it is necessary to stimulate the dorsal columns in order to reach the $A\beta$ primary afferents ordinarily stimulated by TENS. Non-neurogenic stump pain may require treatment by conventional means.

## Central neurogenic pain

Pain following a cerebral vascular accident is usually called thalamic pain, or thalamic syndrome, because the first three cases described all had lesions in the thalamic somatosensory relay nucleus. The advent of computerised axial tomography has confirmed what had long been suspected, that in the majority of cases the lesion is *not* in the thalamus but in pathways leading to or from the somatosensory thalamus. Thus many lesions are found in the postcentral and parietal cortices, and others in the spinothalamic tract[1] in the brainstem. It does not (happily) occur following section of the spinothalamic tract in anterolateral cordotomy, because it is apparently essential that the spino-reticulo-diencephalic ('palaeo-spinothalamic') pathway, inextricably mixed with the direct spinothalamic tract in the spinal cord, be spared.

In any event, clinically the patients are victims of a stroke. There is a tendency for their median age to be younger (about 55) than that of the 'average' stroke patient. Often also the motor effects of the stroke are not particularly severe. In about 50% of cases, the pain is felt from the time that the stroke becomes complete, or very shortly afterwards; in the other half, the burning, sometimes also shooting, pain comes on any time up to 18 months after the cerebro-vascular accident. As in pure motor stroke, the pain may involve a complete body half (or the face on one side and the trunk and limbs on the other), or just the limbs, or just the extremities of the limbs, or the whole or part of a single limb; or a small area on the face, or rarely even on the trunk. The severity of the pain varies from one case to another; it may be little worse than bad 'pins and needles', or it may be excruciating.

There is always an obvious somatic sensory deficit (and also a visual field deficit in true thalamic cases). Although pain only occurs in areas of somatosensory deficit, the two are not necessarily co-extensive: the area of deficit is often larger (but never smaller) than the painful area. It always involves the 'spinothalamic' modalities of temperature and pin-prick (but rarely true tissue-damage pain, such as skinfold pinch); non-spinothalamic modalities may or may not be involved according to the location and extent of the lesion. Allodynia is very common, but not present in every case. Autonomic dysfunction can *always* be detected. The condition is in fact much less rare than is commonly supposed, being commoner than, for example, motor neurone disease.

Treatment is as for other neurogenic pains: peripheral sympathetic blockade where feasible (and as early as possible), combined with medical treatment with tricyclics and anticonvulsants. As is the case in pure motor stroke, pains such as that of frozen shoulder are not uncommon, in addition to neurogenic pain. They must of course be treated in the usual way, by mobilisation, physiotherapy, and NSAIDS.

Central neurogenic pain has occasionally been reported in conditions other than cerebral vascular accident. The commonest are incomplete transection of the spinal cord and multiple sclerosis. In either case, it suffices to be aware that neurogenic pain *can* occur to avoid the mistake of (mis)treating it with conventional analgesics.


## CHRONIC NOCIGENIC PAIN

Because nocigenic, unlike neurogenic, pain interferes with sleep, it is not uncommon for it to present as an emergency, often at highly unsocial hours. The principles of its treatment are well known to every doctor, and there is no intention of repeating them at length here. A few points should, however, be made, particularly with respect to cancer pain:

(1) Never withhold narcotic analgesics for fear of creating dependency or addiction. Apart from the fact that they appear to be rather rare in malignant disease, it hardly matters if they do develop.

(2) Never prescribe analgesics p.r.n., or to be taken 'when the pain comes on'. The aim of therapy is to *prevent* pain from being felt, so dosage must be adjusted to achieve this. Once it has been established how long a particular quantity of analgesic acts for, the next dose must be taken before the first has finished its action. This counsel of perfection is considerably facilitated by the use of slow-release morphine, which frequently need only be taken every 8 or 12 hours.

(3) If bone is thought to be involved, add aspirin (or perhaps diflunisal) to the narcotic. Some authorities consider that aspirin should be given in combination with a narcotic in every case from the very beginning.

(4) Avoid repeated injection of drugs; consider other means of delivery (suppository, epidural/intrathecal catheter) or invasive techniques which may obviate the need for drugs, or at least result in a considerable reduction of dosage: cordotomy, chemical inactivation or destruction of nerve roots or autonomic ganglia; hypophysectomy/pituitary destruction; transcutaneous nerve stimulation. Although these are not emergency procedures, they should be borne in mind even when the patient is seen for perhaps the first time.

## NOTE

1. Thus disposing of the myth that the direct spinothalamic tract is a (or the) 'pain pathway'; and suggesting rather that its function is to *inhibit* pain sensation.

## FURTHER READING

Bond, M.R. (1984) *Pain: its nature, analysis, and treatment*, 2nd edn, Churchill Livingstone, Edinburgh

Bowsher, D. (1985) Pain sensory mechanisms. In: P.J. Vinken, G.W. Bruyn and H.L. Klawans (eds), *Handbook of Clinical Neurology*, Vol. 1, pp. 227–44, Elsevier, Amsterdam

Bowsher, F. (1986) Pain mechanisms in man. *Medical Times (NY)*, *114*, 83–96

Lipton, S. (1979) *Relief of pain in medical practice*. Blackwell Scientific Publications, Oxford/J.B. Lippincott Co., Philadelphia, Pa

Mumford, J.M. (1982) *Orofacial pain*, 3rd edn, Churchill Livingstone, Edinburgh

Swerdlow, M. (ed.) (1988) *Relief of intractable pain*, 4th edn, Elsevier, Amsterdam

# Index

References to Figures and Tables in *italics*